Foundations for a Medical Ethic

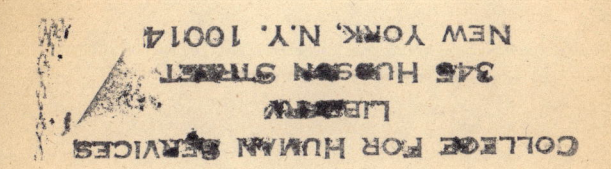

For Dorothy and William, and Brian.

Maurice Reidy

Foundations for a Medical Ethic

*A personal and theological exploration of
the ethical issues in medicine today.*

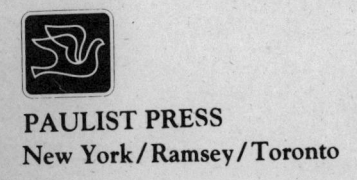

PAULIST PRESS
New York/Ramsey/Toronto

First published 1978 by
Veritas Publications,
7 & 8 Lower Abbey Street
Dublin 1

Copyright © Maurice Reidy 1978

Cover design by Steven Hope

Nihil obstat:
Donal Murray D.D.,
Censor Deputatus

Imprimatur:
 +Dermot,
Archbishop of Dublin,
September 1978

The *nihil obstat* and *imprimatur* are a declaration that a text is considered to be free of doctrinal or moral error. They do not necessarily imply agreement with opinions expressed by the author.

Published in the U. S. A. in 1979
by Paulist Press
Editorial office: 1865 Broadway
 New York, N. Y. 10023
Business office: 545 Island
 Road, Ramsey, N. J. 07446

ISBN: 0-8091-2216-2
Library of Congress
Catalog Card Number: 79-65621

Printed and bound in the U. S. A.

Contents

	Page
Introduction	7
Prologue	9
1 The Human Being	23
2 Sickness and Health	33
3 The Fact of Life	43
4 Consent and Life	51
5 Turning Points	61
6 Distribution and Choice	71
7 Problems of Co-operation	83
8 The Healer	97
Bibliography	103

Introduction

A MEDICAL ethic is principally an attitude, a consciousness, a value-system, which embraces patients, the medical profession, and the whole of society. It is not simply a code that doctors live by, nor even an attitude for which they are primarily responsible. Medicine is the concern of us all, and our doctors and nurses are people of our own culture whose ambitions and responsibilities are enfolded by the ambitions and responsibilities of those whose lives they touch.

The ancient oath of Hippocrates, the father of medical ethics, is a testimony to a sense of trust, a sense of humanity, friendship and family. It pledged to do no harm and to serve only the benefit of the patient. This is the spirit which these pages have tried to capture. They are addressed to our own time from a Christian consciousness that has wanted to bring its own insight to a tradition that is older than the Gospel.

Many issues in medical ethics can only be appreciated from within the day-to-day practice of medicine. In this sense, medical ethics is properly the concern of doctors. They are in a position to judge the moral significance of procedures and investigations, and the professional moralist must be the first to recognise the competence of medicine at this point. He must recognise also the professional ethic which governs standards and relationships within medicine. This book makes no claim that does not respect medical competence in moral matters.

This is a simple book. The word "foundations" is not used pretentiously. It refers to the points of common human concern that underlie the complexities of modern medical questions. The examples and the illustrations reflect only simple human truths, but unless there is a sureness and a confidence at the level of these truths, there is no prospect of pathfinding or of progress in those moments when paths seem to disappear or when a bewilderment of roads seems to offer. The book is intended as an introduction and as a reminder. It opens up in human terms the issues that present themselves in the practice of medicine today, and it provides some points of reference to those simple human facts which ought to govern everything that medicine does.

There is a short reading list at the end. I am heavily indebted to all of the authors who are named there, but there are two books which deserve special mention. *The Patient as Person* by Paul Ramsey has become a classic in its field, and *Aims and Motives in Clinical Medicine*, by Brian P. Bliss and Alan G. Johnson, is the best practical guide I have seen. Ramsey is a moralist and a theologian, and Bliss and Johnson are two practising doctors. In these pages I have sketched some foundations from which these take their strength. Much of what is found here has been taken from them. But the sketch is personal and it includes some detail which they, and perhaps many doctors, would not own. Writing as a priest, it is inevitable that some of the stress that exists within my own faith, especially where it touches on moral development and decline, should find its way into my presentation. Hopefully, this tension will ultimately serve what is best in the care of us all for those to whom we are sent.

I record also the debt I owe to my friends, especially those in the medical and nursing professions, and to my students, whose support and patient criticism has enabled me to write down some of the things we have learned together.

MAURICE REIDY

Prologue

I TRAVELLED to Limerick recently to give a talk on medical ethics. The day was snowy and the passengers on the train shook themselves good-naturedly before sitting down to cast an eye over the evening papers. The weather, as always in Ireland, had introduced us to one another before the journey began. Sitting across from me were a man in his late thirties or early forties and a girl of perhaps twenty. The man was darkly dressed except for a green but conservative tie. There was an air of accomplishment about him, worn lightly. The girl was small, reserved and friendly. She had pleasant brown eyes and her black hair was cropped and boyish. Her clothes were casual—a grey polo necked sweater, matching slacks and a light blue gaberdene coat. At her side was a smart canvas satchel bound in leather. It emerged that the man was a heart specialist and the girl a student nurse. He insisted on first names; he was Henry and she was Barbara.

There were two stories on the front pages that evening, a death sentence and the building of a nuclear reactor. The Government was proposing to build the reactor in anticipation of a greatly increased demand for energy in the years ahead. We soon discovered that Henry was in favour of this, I was somewhat indifferent and Barbara was against it. Henry was convinced that nuclear power was a good thing and that the main worry was one of educating the community to an awareness of the risks to health that were involved, risks that he saw as minimal once the proper steps were taken. I confessed my ignorance of the subject and my mild impatience at the low level of consultation that was going on. Barbara's negative views derived from her concern for ecology in the long term, and these were strongly reinforced by the fact that it was intended to locate the proposed reactor not far from her family home.

We discovered that we were at one mind on the death sentence. We each had received the news with shock and with strong feelings of disapproval. It was difficult to understand how a so-called modern country could presume to enact and execute laws to take life. We shared a common abhorrence of the crime, which had been the killing of a policeman who was acting in the course of his duty. There was a steady opinion in the country which favoured retaining the death penalty for some crimes of violence against the State, and so the law had remained on the statute books, although it seemed to us unlikely that the sentence would be carried out.

We began to discuss the role of law. We were well clear of the city at this stage, and the white countryside seemed like a holiday world. The snow gave the journey a sense of occasion, and the snug atmosphere of the carriage promised to bring the best out of good and genial company. Henry outlined his concept of law. He saw it as a kind of code which gives effect to the will of the people. The ideals and the values of the people, especially their freedoms, need to be enshrined in law so that the society they wish to create and maintain may be understood and supported by all its members. Ultimately, the liberty of every citizen is protected from infringement and violence by the just law.

I took a different line and suggested that ideals and values were not part of the law, not even freedom. For me, the law is the ultimate protection of each individual, whether from his neighbour or from the State. The law guarantees not freedom but justice and fair play. Society is not an association of free individuals who vote laws to guarantee liberty for all; it is itself a kind of organism within which we already find ourselves, some more free than others, and all in need of just treatment.

"Both of you are saying the same thing", said Barbara. Neither Henry nor I would concede this. "As far as I can see," Barbara continued, "each of you could justify a death penalty according to your particular theory, whether on grounds of liberty or on grounds of justice. When everything is boiled down, the real issue is one of bad laws. How do you stop people from making bad laws?" Barbara was earnest. "Who is to guide people? Who is to say what the difference is between justice and injustice? What I would like to know is how to decide who shall be the prisoners and who shall be the court."

It became clear that Barbara was a very moral person for whom right was right and wrong was wrong, regardless of what the law said. This was not Henry's style and when the conversation began to drift in the direction of morality and ethics, he inclined to the view that ethics is an impractical science which was suited only to academic discussion. "It is impossible, especially nowadays, to achieve any kind of ethical consensus, and it is probably unnecessary, as so many of our concepts and presuppositions about man are undergoing profound change. Our generation is producing a new kind of man and a new kind of civilisation, and it is better to hold oneself as open as possible to future development and progress. Ethics, in my experience, is negative and conservative, and it is ill prepared for the kind of debates that are taking place in the world today."

I took this rebuke in good part, and consoled myself that it may have been earned by some of my "flat-earth" friends. I decided to propose a topical parable.

"Imagine a prisoner has been sentenced to death, but the judge gives him one chance of reprieve. The law has been fully complied with, and two citizens are invited to take on themselves the moral decision as to whether the prisoner shall live or die. The two are to meet together for not more than a day, and they must agree one way or the other and issue a statement giving the reason for their decision. It so happens, that of the two citizens chosen, one is in favour of capital punishment and the other is totally opposed to it."

Henry and Barbara accepted the challenge and we began to examine the prisoner's fate. The speed of the train made us lean in towards one another to lend emphasis to our argument. The example was a dilemma, and the truth it illustrated was evident. The two citizens could afford to disagree, each could go his own ethical way. But disagreement was a luxury that the prisoner could not afford. He required agreement as a desperate necessity, and not just agreement, but agreement that capital punishment was morally wrong, and that he must be allowed to live. It was imperative for him that an ethical reason be found, and that both citizens would see that it was certainly valid.

In defence of ethics, I made the point that many of life's problems concern a victim who is waiting for us to decide. If no ethical thinking has been done, and if no sure moral conviction has been formed, then at best, we are acting in the dark, while at worst, we shrug our shoulders and walk away. Many of life's problems already exist before we have begun to think about them; they come along and confront us whether we like it or not.

The conversation was broken for a moment by the arrival of the ticket inspector. We produced our tickets and they were duly punched.

PROLOGUE

Conscience

It was Barbara who resumed, taking up the idea of conscience. "Moral judgements belong to the individual conscience," she asserted, "and without conscience, man is nothing." Henry and I asked her to spell out what she meant by conscience. "Conscience is a kind of intuition", she began, searching for her words carefully. "It is an intellectual and emotional intuition, based on what you think of life and influenced by your family and education."

Barbara was a delicate person, and she had an engaging way of putting things once she warmed to her subject. "It is something that is very deeply rooted, and one cannot always give reasons for judgements of conscience, other than that is what one's conscience says. Most people are aware of certain values, like respect for life, and this shows that conscience is something common between all men, and it shows that conscience is a way of knowing certain deep truths, a way that is very direct and very real." She stopped and considered her words again. "Every country says it respects the rights of conscience, and many people in history have died to preserve these rights. Conscience is part of the human heritage."

Henry weighed this with a smile, drumming his fingers on his knee. He said he was unhappy with the "intuition" aspect of it, and questioned the idea that we should base our deepest convictions on what we had been taught at school or on what our parents said.

"Many people only become moral after they have shaken off their past and their prejudice," I offered. "What about the bigotry between Catholic and Protestant? What about the racial prejudice between black and white?"

Barbara protested that she had not meant to include prejudice and error, and she agreed that moral maturity begins when we start to make our own independent decisions. But she stuck to her point that decision-making rests on values which we have learned to recognise and cherish from our earliest days.

Henry was willing to concede that conscience was one's own personal moral judgement and that it was based on several factors, some of which were laid down in childhood. But he went on to say that, in his opinion, conscience was largely derived from the mental discipline we imposed on ourselves in coming to know things. "Where an important decision is concerned," he said, "we would want to know as much as possible from whatever source, whether science or religion, that could throw light on the matter. That is what conscience is."

Medical Ethics

Encouraged by this development, I thought I would try out some of my ideas for the talk on medical ethics which was to be given later that evening. There were two central points—one was about the spiritual nature of man and the other concerned competence and ethical decisions.

The spiritual idea stressed the personal aspect of the medical relationship. Doctors, nurses and patients are persons primarily, and if the healing process is to succeed it must begin by recognising the personal dimension of those who are involved. The patient is a person, not a medico-social problem. The doctor or nurse is a caring person, not simply a medical agent. The nurse is often closest to the sick person, especially the district nurse in the home situation, and by entering into a prudent companionship and sympathy with the patient and his condition, healing in a "wholesome" sense becomes possible. But when medical persons withdraw from the bedside and take up a position behind the chart or the prescription, they are more likely to be dealing with symptoms than the real illness.

Henry and Barbara shifted restlessly, so I decided to move on quickly. The second point was that an ethical involvement flowed from the personal contact of doctor and patient, that the doctor cannot stand back from ethical implications that are implicit in his treatment. It is not enough to follow one's conscience simply, and to exhort the patient to follow his. The doctor and nurse ought to attempt to identify in a human way with decisions which the patient may be making for the first and only time. This is an extremely delicate matter, and requires competence and sensitivity of a unique kind. Decisions, however difficult, ought not to be left in the air, and patients have a right to expect some help and counsel from the person who brings healing and medical care. Such involvement does not infringe in any way the freedom of conscience of the patient or the doctor, nor need it compromise the role played by the patient's family or clergy. It is a natural follow-through of the personal dimension of medicine.

Barbara was the first to respond to this and she did so by expressing a cautious agreement. The principal difficulty, as she saw it, was that doctors and nurses tended to think medically, not ethically. "That is our job and the way we are trained," she continued, "tends to stress the differences between medical and nursing responsibility rather than the similarities. This may be necessary, but it makes it very difficult for a nurse to enter into an area of responsibility which the doctor would properly consider to be his."

Henry said that the ethical decision and the medical one went together and that doctors would resist the involvement of nurses in medical decisions.

I agreed that the roles of doctors and nurses were different, but I suggested that while it was true that the doctor carried the weight of the medical decision, all parties were equal when it came to moral matters.

Doctor, nurse and patient stand on the same ethical ground. Barbara agreed with this, but felt that the point would need further elaboration before it could be accepted by the medical and nursing professions.

Henry leaned back and said that he had a very fundamental criticism which he would like to share. He spread his hands on his chest and was silent for a moment. He began slowly: "I think that what you are saying is too spiritual and too idealistic. The message of the Churches is too personal, and does not give enough attention to social and political considerations. What is needed is a whole new attitude to the ethics of health care distribution and privilege."

Neither Barbara nor myself had expected this development and we both found ourselves willing to hear more. Barbara asked Henry to go on.

"It seems to me," he said, "that there are two related areas of debate. One concerns the ethics of how we make choices in the allocation of treatment and in the spending of resources. The other concerns the profession directly. If medical training and expertise are to be considered among the goods of society, paid for by society, then what rights does society have in demanding or structuring a return from this asset? What I am asking is this: is medicine a consumer product which follows the free market, or is it something priceless, to be thought of as a kind of gift for which we are all responsible?"

Nobody ventured an answer to this question, but it was clear that Henry was putting his finger on an important ethical issue, perhaps the Cinderella of the moralist's storybook.

The train had come to a standstill at a provincial station, and the voices in the carriage fell to a polite whisper. Henry invited us to the dining-car for coffee. By the time we were seated at the bar, both train and conversation were moving swiftly again. Barbara had raised the nuclear issue as an ethical question. She had been to a meeting on the subject the previous week, and had become an active propagandist against the nuclear project.

"There has been no account taken of the environmental factors that are involved," she said. "On the one side, what about the disposal of nuclear waste, which will remain a threat to all life on the planet for tens of thousands of years? On the other side, have we thought out the implications of making so much energy available, energy that has not been imagined until now? Even if in theory we would say that clean nuclear power was good, could we say that the kind of society that it would generate was right for man? What we should be doing is looking for ways of turning technology in the direction of greater simplicity and independence for each person and family."

Henry said that this line of questioning was similar to one that was going on in medical science. "The revolutionary developments that are taking place in genetics and in replacement surgery are turning our understanding of the human condition upside-down," he said. "But there is no sense in looking at the future as if it were an apple on a forbidden tree. The apple is there and modern man is eating it. Medicine is not going to go backwards, and if we want greater simplicity and more independence, this can only come through scientific achievement properly managed."

I began to say that what we needed was a proper concept of man, one that would include what was essentially human with the changing or evolutionary dimensions of experience. But there was no time to finish the discussion. The train was slowing down as it approached Limerick Junction. We made our way back to our places to collect our baggage and put on our overcoats. Henry said that it was all a matter of how one thought things out, a matter of having the right intellectual framework.

"But it is also a matter of understanding the facts of each situation", added Barbara quickly.

We left the carriage and hurried across the windswept platform to the local train which would take us into Limerick. It was one of those older trains with corridors and separate compartments. When we found a vacant compartment, we moved in and took possession, looking forward to a resumption of our former conversation. We were settling down when a young woman put her head in and asked if there was a seat free. There was a moment's silence before Henry said "Yes, of course". He opened the door fully and she entered. She was attractive, of medium height, a little older than Barbara, and was dressed for the weather in a warm coat, boots and a knitted cap. Henry took her case and put it up on the rack, and she pulled off the cap and shook out her blonde shoulder-length hair. She took the window-seat opposite Barbara who seemed just then to be avoiding her and was looking out at the busy platform.

As I was wondering about this, the young woman caught full sight of Barbara for the first time and a smile of recognition lit her face. "We've met before, haven't we?" she asked, a slight puzzlement behind the smile.

Barbara looked directly at her. "Yes", she said quietly, "I think we have."

Then the woman exclaimed "Of course, I remember now . . . it was just seeing you without your uniform that confused me for a moment. We met in the hospital last week . . . I'm Joan . . . I was in for tests, remember?"

"Indeed I do remember you Joan," Barbara replied, "and I have thought of you since."

"You were very good to me, all of you. I know I may not have shown my appreciation at the time, but the whole thing was just so shattering."

Barbara leaned forward and took Joan's hands in

hers, and said softly "I know, I know . . . it's the hardest thing for a woman to bear."

As she spoke, she glanced at Henry and myself, indicating to Joan by her look that they were not alone. It was a protective gesture and it was obvious to us that whatever the nature of Joan's medical problem, Barbara, who was familiar with it, was not sure whether to accept or stem the tide of revelation that she felt was about to come.

Joan, sensitive to Barbara's concern, smiled calmly, if a little sadly. "I don't mind your friends knowing about it . . . after all, it is a fact of life, isn't it? And I'm not the first, nor will I be the last, to carry this kind of life within me. Perhaps I could talk a little about it, if you don't mind. There have been so many hours alone and in a little while I will be meeting my family."

Barbara's nursing instinct recognised the possible value of this. She was conscious by now that Henry and I were prepared to be willing listeners, and she turned to us and said "Joan is expecting a baby, and she has had very bad news about it."

Henry and I looked at Joan sympathetically . . . was she going to lose it?

"No," declared Joan, "I am not going to lose it although for several days I wished it were lost, gone, taken away. The results of the tests have shown that it is deformed".

Shocked, Henry and I looked pityingly at her. We were helplessly unable to find anything to say.

She looked steadily back at us. "I was shattered. I was sick at the thought of having conceived a disaster. I knew there might be a problem, but when the doctor gave me the news that it was deformed, everything in me collapsed. Everything in me rejected it . . . I hated what they told me was in my womb . . . this couldn't happen to me and I didn't care how or where it would go as long as it was gone."

The train was on its way and the carriage rocked uncomfortably from side to side. How different an experience for us was the human story that was unfolding, from the stimulating and provocative discussion which had passed the first part of the journey.

Joan gazed out through the window at the wintry landscape. "I will never forget the hell of those first couple of days. I couldn't face the journey home. How could I bring this news home to my family? I dragged myself back to the hospital, not knowing what I would ask for. I could not cope with a future which included what was growing inside me."

Barbara crossed to sit beside her and put her arm on her shoulder in a wordlessly comforting gesture. Joan rested against her. Then the smile came back.

"A funny thing happened to me going up the hospital steps." She turned to Barbara. "You know the way there are always half a dozen mums waiting for taxis, holding their precious little bundles, cooing over them and smiling proudly at everyone who passes in and out?"

Barbara nodded, "You'd think there wasn't another baby like them in the world."

"That's exactly what I thought," said Joan "as I watched one mother cuddle her beautiful, healthy child to her breast, and overheard her whisper to it. The thing is, that's what I thought about my own baby. I realised, watching that mother, that one day, my child, my poor broken child could lie in my arms, and I, it's mother, could give it all the love in the world. For the first time I thought of it as flesh of my flesh, and it's very infirmity made it even more precious. I would give it everything that I could. I felt a great sense of possessiveness take over and replace all the rejection. I wanted this child and I wanted to cherish it as completely as possible."

PROLOGUE

Joan sat back in her seat, closing her eyes as the memories of the past few days passed before her. There was a silence except for the rattling of the wheels.

"Don't think I'm unaware of what I am facing. I know there will be sadness. I also know that what I am saying and feeling now may not always be said and felt in this way. But I know that what I am doing is right. The despair is gone, and the peace and acceptance and the bond that I feel now tells me that this love and caring will always be true, no matter how it feels. I never thought that anyone, least of all my own deformed infant, could claim me in this way. Perhaps God was looking for a parent for this very special child and he has chosen me."

Again there was silence. What could one say? She had shared her agony and was now saying "Yes" in a way which would seem incomprehensible to many. Her strength and truth were revealed in the next words she spoke.

"I don't mind admitting that I would have preferred a miscarriage to bearing a deformed or retarded baby. In the light of what I've said that may seem strange, but do we not often say when someone we love has died 'it is better that way, we would not have wished them to live on'. Yet we do not want them gone, and certainly we would never kill or take their life away."

It seemed so simple and so prophetic. She had shared her sense of being blessed, and there was nothing we could say.

1 The human being

IMAGINE THE ROUTINE preparations in a hospital theatre as the surgical team await the arrival of the victim of a traffic accident. Nobody knows the identity of the patient. Each one takes up his position. The doors open, the trolley is wheeled in and the patient is placed on the operating table. The anaesthetist looks down and sees there the face of her own son. The victim is no longer a patient, the anaesthetist is no longer a doctor. The son is unconscious, and nobody has noticed the horror behind the mother's mask.

Modern medicine is built on facts. Around facts are gathered knowledge, expertise, experience, skill. The whole is clinical and dispassionate, a wonder of civilisation. But the one supreme fact which bears upon the anaesthetist is a fact of which none of the team is aware, a fact of no medical importance, a fact which belongs to the realm of the subjective rather than the objective world. Had there been another person in her place, this overwhelming fact would not have been present. And yet this one fact, that the patient is her own son, has transformed the routine reality of accustomed science into the most agonising professional and personal crisis she has ever faced.

It is not simply a question of shock, nor of fear. It is rather that the whole fiction associated with medical technology has broken down. She is not confronted with a pulse-rate, but with the heartbeat of her son. The success of the operation depends on each member of the team seeing only the narrow range of bodily and physiological functions presented on the table. That is the only objectivity the team can know; that is the only reality it can afford to see. And the reality that the mother sees blinds her. Had she seen nothing, she might have carried on.

We can easily make the mistake of thinking that the only facts are objective ones, that is, the ones that are observable and measurable. The facts that we classify as subjective may be more real. Reality has an infinite range. If we consider the whole of our lives and the wide range of our personhood, we realise that it is the subjective facts that are the essential ones. Nobody cares about a hand or an eye when the whole self is in the balance. And what is the self, the person? It is not something that can be seen on the operating table, certainly not anything that can be touched with syringe or scalpel.

Subjectivity and Man

Subjectivity is the heart of the human paradox. The human being belongs to everything that biology is, and yet transcends biology totally. The development of all life, from the most primitive of cells millions of years ago, has led to the emergence of one species that is utterly different. Like the plants, this species has growth and decline, and like the animals of every kind, it has feeling and intelligence. But unlike anything else that our planet has brought forth, this species, man, can reflect and know truth. The planet Earth has produced life which in turn has become thought. It would never have happened if it could never have happened. Our world has come from matter to mind.

The boy on the table has a slim chance of survival. It depends on whether or not the surgeon can repair vital tissue quickly. Tissue: there's a word to play with, stuff, condition, time. Like a telephone engineer, the surgeon handles cables small and large and of various colours. The conversation that jumps along the lines is not the engineer's concern, just that the condition, the time and the conjunction are right. As the minutes pass, the boy begins to die. A person, a world, is poised on the conjunction of tissue. Like the sailor lost at sea, a world flickers, cut off by time and by conditions from another world struggling by every means to come and save. When the tissue dies, a world is gone.

Whether one takes the long view, standing back from everything and looking at mankind as a species, or whether one stands close and studies the individual person, one is confronted with a reality that defies total understanding. There is something of a mystery on hand. It is wise to select various aspects of the human being which we can understand fully, when by so doing, we can apply in a helpful way the knowledge that we gain. But equally, it is foolish to pretend that when we have successfully isolated the working of tissue, or the patterns of the mind, that we are then in possession of a total understanding of man. It may be useful to term our practical knowledge as objective, but it is unhelpful and misleading to suppose that what we thus call objective is all that there is. The fact that the boy is the mother's son is an objective fact, and to her the subjective relationship with her son is the one fact which takes precedence over all others.

What is objectivity? It may be said that thought and friendship are objective. Human life creates a new objectivity in the world which is infinitely more important than the objectivity of the physical conditions on which it is dependent, more important than the body and the language through which love is learned and expressed. The body is precious, but the man is everything. Human life is the experiment of the human spirit. It is the growth and strengthening of the sinews of parental and marital love, the maturing of community fellowship and trust. We may prefer to term our different understandings of the human spirit as subjective, and we may prefer to call the human world which we ourselves create as persons a subjective world. But we cannot mean by that that its existence is less real. The world of meaning and of love is precisely the human achievement, the world we are born to sustain. The world of relationships and of understanding is man's domain.

Objectivity and God

What is the significance of God? Is God a fact? Religion is something that we tend to classify as subjective, but here too our use of words can be misleading. It is true to say that all men, of religious belief and of none, must concede that their understanding of God conditions their understanding of everything. That is a fact. If one does not believe in God, then one has a different apprehension of the world from the person who does believe. Furthermore, what one apprehends of the world is directly influenced by the apprehension one has of other realities. Like the mother and the son, the fact of how one sees has a vital bearing on what one sees. It is a fact that faith in God makes a profound difference.

We might ask where God is to be found. The concept of trust, or faith, is used to describe a state of mind that comes to know God. The question as to where God is is not as different as we may suppose from the question which seeks to penetrate the secret of man. Where is the human person? How does one touch a person? In a mysterious way the person pervades the body, is manifest when we encounter one another, is hidden when we try to be more exact. The human person is to be found in silence and in words. God is quite distinct from us and from the universe, and yet he pervades everything mysteriously. The trust with which we intimately know one another is like the simplicity, humility and faith in which we can discover God. He creates the universe, and when each of us comes into the world we find his simplicity already there. The Christian faith discovers God in silence and in words.

In his words, God appears as one who is conversant with every aspect of human life. His message is one of compassion and encouragement. He calls men to be with him, to "overcome" the world. His human creature is expected to be strong in heart and to transcend the contradictions of life. The vision of man that emerges from the pages of scripture is one of courage, dignity and infinite worth. If God has a vision of man, then Christians will find their own vision and understanding of humanity in his. If we know that the hairs on every head are numbered, that no sparrow falls to the ground unheeded, then we know something of the subjectivity of God. We know something of how he sees every creature, sick and well. We know something of what he sees in every person, young and old. And we know too that whatever healing we can bring to flesh and blood makes more sense than we could have imagined. We know that God is a profoundly grateful parent.

The problem of pain

There are some things that we must try to understand, if not completely, at least correctly. Why does the parent permit pain? This problem can be made more difficult by preconceived ideas about God and the world. If we do not listen carefully to his word, we may find ourselves projecting onto him needs and fears that are characteristic of the child, not the adult. We will find ourselves making God in our own image and likeness, and we will be frustrated with our invention. Children tend to project their fantasies onto their parents. This does not contradict the fact that we are born of mothers and fathers; one could argue that it confirms it. We must come to know life and its creator on their own terms, not ours. The real God respects us, and if we listen we will learn that life is infinitely worthwhile, despite the problems.

A first observation about pain is that it is in some sense necessary. If we did not feel our fingers burn in a flame, then we would be prey to every danger. We would lack the most elementary warning system. It is also necessary in the sense that it is part of our condition. Because we are physical, our organs can malfunction and our limbs can break. Because we share the biological world, we share a world in which progress and decline induce new states and developments. In simple terms, our life is an organic one and it is vulnerable and impermanent of its nature. It replaces itself and dies.

A second observation about pain is that it is relative. The soldier who loses a leg in battle may smile at the doctor and consider himself lucky to be alive, while the guest with a toothache may be dejected and consider his day ruined. Many things that are wrought with pain become a joy we would not change for the world. We see this every day in pregnancy and in childbirth. And a couple whose marriage has been scarred by years of illness may find that their love has now achieved a richness which comes only to the few. Would they prefer it to have been otherwise, if it seems their love would have been otherwise too? None of these considerations is meant to justify pain. They remind us that pain is, like other things in life, a condition despite which men and women flourish.

But what about pain that is manifestly pointless? In a strange way, this is a Christian question and a Christian contradiction at the same time. It is important to realise that only the person who believes in God asks this question. The person who believes there is no God believes there is no question; pointless pain is a simple fact. This is crucial. Only the non-believer resigns the right to be dissatisfied. Pointless pain stops our world, we throw away everything in the struggle to be free again. It is a hook cast into the mouth of life.

I believe that people who honestly ask this question

in a spirit of prayer will always receive an answer, perhaps an answer that only they themselves can understand, an answer that comes from the silence of God. It may be an answer which changes their assumptions about life, perhaps one that helps them to change themselves. One meets seriously ill patients who have begun to find the answer. Often their difficulty is to persuade us who are well to accept what they can now accept. One also meets patients who are damaged and embittered, patients for whom pain continues to be a disaster in every sense, because they have been unable or unwilling to seek or find any deeper understanding. It is a great mistake to assume too readily any general or theoretical explanation of suffering. It is as unhelpful and unreal to dismiss pain, as it is to glorify it. Those who stand by ought to be compassionate and silent, unless they themselves know the truth of what they say. Pain is mysterious, and it belongs to the region of darkness between each man and God.

Christians have always seen God as a kind of doctor. Jesus spoke of himself as a physician who comes not to those who are well, but to the sick. Answers about suffering are to be found in God's understanding of human life and maturity. Jesus of Nazareth was not a fantasy figure; he was a youthful artisan who reached into the pith of each life that encountered him and tried to draw forth reluctant creatures who thought they had grown enough. I believe he speaks to us through the maturity and silence of every patient who suffers.

Heaven and earth

The artisan God befriends us to make us like himself. What does he see in us? Why does he make himself vulnerable to our rejection? It can only be because he sees in each of us what the mother sees in her son.

What does the mother see? She sees someone whose life is part of her own, whose existence has been given and nurtured by herself. She sees one who was totally dependent on her, one to whom she has committed the direction her own life has taken. She sees someone she has taught to be a man. She looks beyond the confidence and the fear, the gift and the limitations, the success and the failure. She sees the unique, irreplaceable, wonderful person of her own child. She loves every part of him, great and small. She loves the hand, the fingers, the wrist. She loves to look and to touch and to hold. She holds him to her face.

She loves his body and is distressed by his illness. Yet the ugliness of injury does not diminish that love, it intensifies it. She desires him to be whole again and until that moment comes, he enjoys a special and privileged claim on her. She cannot feel any differently from the way she does, and he needs nothing else than to be who he is.

Again, there is a sense of paradox. It is the paradox of time, of detail, of earth. Time is a moment in eternity, detail is a fragile circumstance in an infinite universe. Yet time is precious and our circumstances are all that we have. They will not come again. Have we been born to live a healthy life simply, and join our fathers in the grave? The length of all time and the breadth of all space remind us that the present will soon be gone. Does sickness matter? Was it good to have been born?

How does one measure the good life? What profits a man? What does the mother wish most for her son? What does the mother dread most for her son? When would she judge it better that he had not been born? Illness is not the greatest tragedy, nor is death. This is the great paradox, that we can lose everything and be still stronger, we can possess everything and be lost. In sickness we can possess our humanity more richly than we possessed it in health. And we believe that when we die, we meet God face to face, we discover the infinite

THE HUMAN BEING

dimensions of truths we glimpsed in life. We discover that love is what God is.

The adventure of mankind is in its beginnings. We have arrived at an apprehension of what is spiritual. Which of us can say that this is our own achievement? Which of us can say that we have made the world, or even that we have made ourselves? The same One that has given us the truth we already perceive, has promised an eternity of fulfilment to his burdened creatures. We cannot deny the future, we who have received everything that the present is. We cannot deny heaven, when we have to admit that earth already exists.

A young woman nurses her father. What does he hear when she says "Dad"? What does he see when their eyes meet? She is the woman to whom everything is given. She is the softness in whom all bitterness disappears, the mystery in which all hard edges are made smooth. Everything that is womanly he loves in her. Everything that is manly in himself seems to take second place. Does he hear his own name being called? Does he recognise in her a life that was his to give? He may be tempted to think that he sees in her what is best in himself, but this is only a temptation. How could this woman be a reflection of him? How can any man give himself a daughter? The love of the father goes out to something that is greater than himself. It reminds him of his powerlessness and of the grace he has been given. And there is no end to grace.

Is this the world that we call subjective? Surely this is the real world, these are the real values which medical science is given to serve and sustain. We are in the presence of man. Our understanding of the human person must look to him as he has been created to be. A fictional world of tissue and function would not be worth the effort if it were not pervaded by the dignity of man. The true object of medical care is the human being.

2 Sickness and health

IT IS SAD to meet devoted parents who are worried about what will happen to a sick child after they themselves are gone. It is a natural worry. Doctors, when they are treating patients who are mentally ill, will sometimes wonder if they are acting in the best interest of the patients, or if they are acting in the interest of society. It seems that the interest of patients and of society do not always run together. Families do not always recognise fully the claim made upon them by those who are ill. Society can unreasonably demand the removal of the sick, and charge medical care with making up for what is wanting in a fast and complex world. But medical care, and the expensive outlay which it involves, cannot be expected to provide by itself the affirmation and acceptance which are the real price of healing.

A doctor may decide that a particular patient will be helped by being taken into institutional care. Such care may succeed only by imposing a strict regime on the patient, a regime which may include sedation as a normal feature of daily routine. It is not in dispute that the discipline of hospital life, medication and nursing care are indispensable elements in the battle against sickness and disease. But the question arises as to whether this treatment deprives this patient of the opportunity of expressing and becoming his true self, of discovering his own personality. Is the organism that is human society doing its best for this patient? Without having to appeal to a mythical life of nature, we know that if our society were more simple and hospitable there would be room in the world for many who are slow and who need to be free.

This same kind of question can be posed about the prescription of drugs. How often is the treatment of patients, whether at home or in hospital, governed more by the pressures of time and life which bear upon the doctor, than by the needs of the persons to whom he has been called? Ultimately it is futile to expect that patients and doctors will find conditions in life that are perfect, but we ought not to attempt to provide limbo-type solutions to problems that have their origin not only in those who are sick, but in those who are well.

The doctor and the nurse play an indispensable part in the healing process. It is a medical and personal role, and one which needs to be filled out by other persons, especially the relatives and friends of the patient. The sick need above all the ministry and the encouragement that comes from those who are well. Sickness, like symptoms, cannot be compartmentalised. This is more evident in the case of mental illness, where the greatest demands are made on faithful medical and family care. Medicine is not an end in itself, its purpose is to return the patient to a state of health whenever this is possible, and if society is to be faithful, it must welcome and make place for every patient, it must be available to the weakest in a way which will allow them to be themselves.

Ideally speaking, there should be no conflict between a patient and his environment; each should be adequate to the other. But this is not the way of life. In many situations, not all of them concerned with sickness, doctors are faced with conflict, and pressed for solutions which they know to be inappropriate. Medical solutions can be related to symptoms merely, and not to the underlying problem. A wife may request that her fertility be supressed because of the irresponsibility of her busband, but is her problem a medical one? Would a sterilising intervention do any good against the hurt that irresponsibility will continue to inflict? Would it make conjugal intimacy an act of love? The doctor rightly asks himself how he is to act in the best interest of this patient, and not simply in the interest of her inadequate environment.

Ethical questions

What is the purpose of medicine? Is it to solve life's problems and compensate for our inadequacies? Perhaps its role is to stimulate us when we need a push, or to pacify us if we move too fast? Should it attempt to make us better people, or more useful?

We should ask who are the doctors and the nurses. Are they the graduates of medical and nursing schools, or the administrators of our hospitals and health services? Are they the shareholders, managers or employees of companies which produce medical goods? Who else is responsible? Who else is answerable for our patients?

And who are the patients? Who are the sick among us? Certainly the physically and mentally infirm, and most of the rest of us from time to time, when need arises. What kind of need? How do we know?

How do we know, indeed? And where does the moralist come in? Who is he and what right has he to be heard? He speaks for nobody but himself, yet he questions in the name of his own humanity. He puts the human questions that suggest themselves behind every civilised endeavour. And medicine is full of human questions. As a theologian he tries to relate the human questions to God's word.

The answers to ethical questions are to be found in an understanding of the human task. The human task is what we have been born for, the realisation of the gift of ourselves. To appreciate that gift we need a concept of man; we need to know something about freedom, about love, about responsibility, about goodness. The human task belongs to a world which seems to lack these qualities as much as it possesses them.

It is a task to be undertaken by ourselves; nothing we can invent can do it for us. It is done in sickness and in health, and when illness slows us in our tracks medicine helps us to resume as best we can. But it is we ourselves who resume, it is we ourselves who take up the reins of freedom and of love.

We need a concept of ourselves which includes both change and continuity. We live at a time when customs and expectations from life and the world are undergoing profound change. Yet it is the same man, the same patient, the same open-handed sinner who needs to be renewed and to be saved.

We need a concept of health. Until we have understood the human task we cannot know what health is. It is through our perception of man that we can know when he is sick; it is through our perception of responsibility and goodness that we can heal and comfort him. Health takes us to the heart of medicine.

The medical indication

The best interest of the patient refers primarily to his good health, and it is not as easy as it seems to give an exact definition of this. The concepts of health and sickness are so familiar and so obvious, that we hardly ever question them. They depend on one another for their meaning and it is impossible to describe one without having in mind the other. Whatever is considered important in our picture of man will find its way into our definition of health, and this can include very different qualities, such as physical strength and self-respect.

Somewhere in between sickness and health, occupying ambiguous territory which is claimed by each side, is the concept of handicap. A person who is blind, or lame or mentally deficient, ought to be considered healthy, and ought always to be treated as such, within the limitations imposed by his condition.

There is a truth in the obviousness of the concepts of health and sickness, and in their ambiguity. There is a profound moral truth in their distinctness. It is precisely this distinctness which guides medicine and shapes its task. If there is no proper perception of health, then the goal of medicine is obscured. If there is no perception of health, then all human difficulty is in danger of being seen as a kind of sickness, and problems that are human begin to look towards medicine for their solution. But to introduce institutional care, or drugs, or surgery, into the area which is properly occupied by mature, if assisted, human response, is to undermine the foundations of human living.

The problems of those who are well must be faced from a standpoint of health, with the strength that comes from conviction and the support of friends. Medicine aims to restore health and prevent illness, and if it has no adequate means of distinguishing one from the other, it may begin to supplant health with false support, and induce illness by depriving patients of the challenge to be themselves.

Before treatment to induce a change in the condition of a patient is initiated, the doctor ought to ask "What is this condition?" If the answer to this question falls outside the definition of illness, then he ought to ask what he is trying to change, and why.

These questions highlight the significance of a true medical indication, that is, the presence in the patient of a sick condition. Whether at the level of the individual, or of society as a whole, it is the business of medicine to prevent and cure illness, to maintain health. Gratuitous interference or manipulation falls outside the scope of medical science, whether it relates to the healthy conditions of patients or of whole populations, whether it has been requested in the name of knowledge or of convenience.

The distinction between health and sickness provides the first and most fundamental moral insight into the medical task. A medical indication is one which calls for medical intervention on its own terms. The ancients formulated this same insight in the injunction "do no injury". To induce change in healthy persons is to run the risk of doing them an injury, and may deprive them of the substance of the human task. Life may have fewer problems when freedom or fertility has been removed, but what does that prove?

Medicine needs a firm concept of the healthy man and woman, a concept which includes vulnerability, weakness, handicap and old age. It needs a concept of man which preserves the dignity of the person and of the human condition in each phase of life and in each of life's situations. Personal, social and political indications are the business of persons, society and the State, and they do not as such demand or require medical assistance.

Medical indications provide an essential sense of direction in an age when science has embarked on a programme of experiment and control in service of the human condition. Every hospital and every medical school wants to be part of this endeavour. But innovation which is not grounded in a sympathetic respect for healthy manhood and womanhood will probably do more injury than good. It may make the mistake of attempting to alter what is human, rather than assisting it. Medical technology may soon be able to allow us to run faster by replacing our natural organs with fabricated machines, but what becomes of the contest of true athletes? The hundred metres is a human test, not simply a test of speed. Manipulation may be able to induce changes which make the sexes more alike, but what is to become of the encounter of men and women? resuscitation and transplant surgery can postpone death, but what is the point of postponement if there is no real assistance given to the human task of living and dying? All of us who owe our life and fitness to the expertise of medicine are rightly grateful; we are grateful for having been healed, and for having been helped to live again our human response to life. That response will not be threatened by the limitations inherent in human living, nor by death when its time has come, but it may be removed altogether in those from whom the human foundation of dignity, freedom and the ability to love and to die has been taken away.

This is not the place for a blue-print of a healthy society. But criticism there must be where the pressures of work and modern domestic hardships are pushing men and women more and more towards a medical re-fabrication of their lives and persons.

The concept of totality

The concept of totality is an important adjunct to the medical indication. It attempts to view the patient in an overall perspective which will facilitate medical and moral decisions. It is inseparable from the condition and the person.

At the simplest level it views the human body as a totality, and permits treatment which may be painful or injurious in the short term, but which contains a promise of return to health. For this reason a limb may be amputated or a function supressed, if it directly threatens the health of the whole body. At a more complex level it views the human person as a totality, and permits treatment which may be injurious to the patient in some respect, but which is justified by the need to contain and control an otherwise unmanageable pathological condition. This is an extremely delicate matter, particularly in the case of severe mental illness when a patient may need to be committed to long-term hospital and institutional care.

At this more complex level the principle of totality may also permit treatment which is injurious to the body considered in itself, but which is therapeutic to a pathological condition which is present in another person. For this reason a healthy person may donate a kidney where there is just cause. Another application of the concept of totality at this level would allow the supression of fertility where the procreative faculty had become impaired in a truly pathological way. In this case appeal is made to the total person as a spouse, and supression of fertility is justified on the basis that, by reason of its pathological association, it has become an obstacle to the fulfilment of the human task in marriage.

Fertility has become one of the principal areas of medical and moral controversy in our day. Sexual intercourse is seen mainly as a function of love and appreciation between men and women. At the medical level the procreative role has been put in question, and at a moral level, both procreation and the marital setting of intercourse have been widely challenged as guiding principles of behaviour. Yet, both medically and morally, the concept of totality would seem to demand a respect for all the dimensions of human sexuality. There is a love dimension and a procreative dimension in the sexual faculty; it is unitive and procreative. A medical ethic which would depart from this most human evidence can hardly bear promise of wholeness or health. And the fulfilment of persons that is betokened by the unitive and procreative faculty of sexuality belongs to an atmosphere, an understanding, a commitment, in which two persons accept and cherish the totality of person and life in one another.

As it applies in medicine, the concept of totality depends on the presence of a true medical indication. Be it the cure of illness, or the maintenance of health, the course of treatment relates directly to the pathology that threatens.

The concept of totality demands that each human subject be seen in its totality, and that each party to a medical or a moral conflict enjoys full and appropriate rights of medical care. Traditionally, the purposes of medicine have been given as the cure of illness, the saving of life, the relief of pain. In all of these ends the doctor and the nurse serve the human task of the patient and their decisions are fully informed when taken in this total perspective. There are no categories of illness, or health, or handicap which make a subject less human, or which confer rights on one patient at the expense of another. The unborn and the aged have an equal claim to be considered in their totality.

The patient as person

There is a further question which admits the doctor to the best interest of his patient. This is: "Who is the patient?" The answer to this question reveals the person, and the human context of friendship and family to which he belongs. The desire to banish illness must not allow itself to be infected with an indifference to those who are ill, and to their world. Not just sickness, but insensitive medicine can undermine humanity. The slave-traders of bygone days examined the human beings on offer at the auction, and looked at their teeth, their hands and their feet. An insensitive medicine takes account only of the condition, and bypasses the person.

The medical task is more than the banishment of illness, it is the healing of the patient. The patient is healed to the extent to which he is helped to resume the human task, to take up again his position in his world. This cannot be done unless respectful contact is maintained with the person and with his environment, and unless there is a sympathetic understanding and encouragement mediated both by medicine and by the patient's world.

Patients ought not to be isolated, nor ought we leave

the problems of the sick to medicine simply. Doctors and nurses do not perform their duty in quarantine, but in the healthy world in which the patient is ill. If the world is not well there is something out of joint; the impossible is being attempted. Medicine belongs to a caring world whose business is to seek the recovery of the patient. If everyone were sick, medicine would not make sense.

The recovery of the patient restores him to the human task, to the call of responsibility and love which life addressed to us. That task can know joy and pain, fulfilment and frustration, success and failure. Medicine does not take the sharp edge from life, it helps us to meet that edge with courage when only illness makes us weak.

By asking "Who is the patient?" the doctor puts himself in the presence of the persons he serves.

By his knowledge of the medical indication and of the person of the patient, the doctor prepares himself for a decision concerning the correct treatment that is to be given. It may be that the full measure of institutional, medical or surgical care is required. But it may also be that this is too much, and if this treatment is prescribed, medicine will have erred by excess, and the world will have erred by defect. If this is true of the care of mental illness, where the human dilemma is cast in greater relief, it is true of all medical care. Medicine can overkill, and we can feel ourselves to be exonerated from our own human task, the task of those who are well to care for our sick. As in the case of the woman who is worried by her husband's irresponsibility, there are several parties to the problem. Her interest needs to be consulted not only by the doctor, but by her husband. The human task requires that we address ourselves to the whole patient, the total person, and that we do so as whole people ourselves.

3 The fact of life

THE NURSE takes the patient's wrist in her hand and looks steadily at her watch. At the tips of her fingers the heart beats. She knows that all is well, the pulse is right. She is an expert at reading the signs. If the pulse is too fast, or too slow, the patient is in trouble. And if there is no pulse, he is probably dead.

What are the signs of life? There is perhaps no more controversial area in medicine today than this. The obvious facts which guided judgements about death and life in the past have now been overturned. A stopped heart need not be the end, and where are we to locate the beginning? It is possible to restart and maintain the activity of heart and lungs and it is possible to monitor the first divisions of cells in a test tube. Is it possible to pinpoint the moment of death or to say that at a particular moment in time, a new person has arrived on the scene?

In ordinary everyday practice, two kinds of cases are likely to present themselves with particular urgency. The first is when a serious abnormality has been detected in early pregnancy and when doctor and patient need to know if the foetus is already human. The second is when a serious illness or accident has brought life to an end and there is a demand for organ donation; doctor and next of kin need to know whether or not the patient is already dead. The signs of life, whatever we judge them to be, indicate two things, one is the fact of life, the other is the condition of that life. Medical ethics is concerned with how we interpret the fact of life, and with how we respond to its condition.

Beginning and end

When does life begin? What are the signs? We might begin by examining the different physical stages of early development. Does life begin at fertilisation, or does it begin some days later at implantation? Some would suggest that it does not begin until some time after implantation when the possibility of twinning has passed. Some would delay some weeks until familiar human features begin to appear, or even later, until the time when electrical activity can be detected in the brain. Some would hold that human life begins only when the foetus becomes viable, when it is capable of sustaining its own life outside the womb.

The possibility of twinning deserves special attention. This is when a division takes place that creates identical twins. Do two lives begin then? Or does a second life begin where there had been only one? Until it has been made clear that we ought not to consider the first organism as a parent, from which a twin has now been born, we must presume that life has begun at fertilisation. The difficulty with all the other stages is that they seem to be arbitrarily chosen. Except for fertilisation, and for the division that creates an identical twin, there is no moment in which what is already present enters a substantially new phase. Before fertilisation there was nothing, whereas after it, each stage is a natural development that grows from the stage preceding it. There is a progress that begins at a certain point and continues thereafter. The stage of viability offers least help because it is itself so mobile, and so dependent on outside factors. Viability comes progressively earlier according as appropriate medical care becomes more sophisticated. Whether or not life has begun is hardly indicated by our own ability to cope with it.

Sometimes the question is approached from a personal angle. When are we dealing with a human person?

Is it before birth, or on the occasion of birth? As with viability, it is difficult to see what difference birth makes. The moments before and the moments after birth tell us nothing new about the personhood of the child. It would be more logical to appeal to the time when child and mother can recognise one another, when the little human being can relate to other people and become aware of itself. Another landmark in this series would be the age of reason, when the child begins to think. Further on is adolescence, when the adult begins to emerge and take possession of self and life, or indeed one might go on until marriage, parenthood or full maturity. But it would be manifestly absurd to withold recognition of human life until then.

And what are the signs of death? At what moment can we say that life has ended? Opinions about death are also based on both personal and physiological criteria. There are those who would suggest that life has ended once the capacity for relationships has been lost. This might be when suffering has made the burden of life seem insupportable. A variant of this is the suggestion that life ends when reason is impaired or when senility sets in. The loss of the intellectual faculties would be taken as an indication of the end of life. Clearly if this kind of thinking were to take hold, many patients who suffer an intellectual handicap would never be permitted to live in the first place. It is a fact that many people are already firmly disposed towards termination in the womb of life that is deformed.

More familiar to us are the physiological criteria. These have traditionally been the spontaneous cessation of heart and lungs, when circulation stops and the patient breathes his last. They have provided good and trusted service until the present day. But medical knowledge and skill have now transformed our approach to these criteria, because it is clear that death does not infallibly attend these events. If something is done, death may be put off until another day.

This is only one side of the problem. If heart and lungs can be manipulated independently of death, then may death not sometimes already be present, even when the heart is made to beat and the lungs are made to breathe? If the heart's stillness is no longer a sign of death, then its beat may not be a sign of life. May a patient be pronounced dead, even when circulation and ventilation are maintained?

It is asserted now that a certain criterion of death is the complete cessation of electrical activity in the brain, when this is accompanied by the spontaneous cessation of heart and lungs. The irreversible cessation of electrical activity in the brain may be safely verified under certain conditions. It is possible to monitor this activity while heart and lungs are being artificially maintained, and once life in the brain terminates finally, then it is a simple matter to verify the termination of heart and lungs by withdrawing artificial support. When this is done, the body may be put back again on artificial ventilation and circulation, and even though the lungs breathe and the heart beats, it is clear that death has taken place. Life is not being supported, but a corpse is being held in readiness so that an organ may be transplanted and used again.

But can it be said that the cessation of brain activity is the moment of death? What medicine has provided is a new way of knowing if death has already taken place. Naturally death announces itself within a very short time, and so does life. The moment belongs to God.

Theology and medicine

Death is a metaphysical event. It cannot be seen, nor heard, nor touched. It is the same with the beginning of life. One moment we are in the presence of life, another moment we are not. We cannot see a spiritual event, although we can know when it has happened. To understand the fact of life, we need to reflect on the mystery of man.

Theology and medicine each contribute to this task. The different role of each must be correctly perceived. Both are anchored firmly in the world of human experience, one to interpret what is to be known of God and the human spirit, one to investigate what is to be known of the body and the mind of man. There is a natural overlap, a meeting-place in which each learns from the other, and there is a province which is proper to each. Some of medicine's most difficult ethical decisions occur within this overlap.

Theology properly describes the soul as that aspect of man which is spiritual and transcendent, and which survives the body in death, even though we believe that the body too will live again in a way which we cannot now understand. But theology ought not to create the impression that the soul precedes the body, or that there is a moment when the soul joins the body. Theology cannot identify any moment in life when a soul is "infused". To attempt to do so is to misunderstand the concept of soul. Theology reflects on the spiritual dimension of human life, and this is indivisible. All human life is spiritual, all human life has a soul.

Medicine properly describes the body as that aspect of man which is subject to physical growth and decline. It ought not to suggest that the body precedes the soul, or that it survives it. Underlying such suggestions may be concepts of "sub-human" or "less human". But there is no imaginary line below which our humanity disappears. Nor is there any choice about who is human and who is not, whether in medicine or ethics or politics. Man is a unity of body and soul, a unity which is indivisible in life. That unity is present in every moment, including the first and the last. There is no such stage as "half dead" or "nearly dead". We are always fully

alive, or we are gone. We can say with certainty that
a deceased person is departed or gone, but we cannot
say that an embryonic person has "not yet arrived".
There is no human life that has not yet arrived.

Medicine, not theology, can tell us when life has
begun, and when life has ended. Theology, not medicine,
can tell us about the spiritual significance of human
life. There is no way that life that has begun, or life
that is not yet ended, can be shown to be other than
human. Difficult as decisions can be within the overlap
of theology and medicine, if our theoretical understanding
is sound, then we have a foundation from which
conscience may more freely decide what ought to be
done.

The condition of life

The signs of life tell us about its condition. It may
be ill or handicapped, or deformed. And they give us
some indication of how we may respond to that condition.
It ought to be a positive response, even though
this may represent a challenge and a threat to our
own aspirations. A positive response from the parents
of the deformed child is no easy thing for anyone to
command. A positive response to the comatose patient
can be unnerving for the doctor who counts the minutes
as another patient waits for his chance to be saved.

But every human subject is deserving of appropriate
medical care and support in his own right. We must
ground our response in this fundamental fact. There
can be no distinction between persons when it comes
to supporting life. We are not empowered to sit in
judgement on specimens that are less than perfect.
We are not empowered to end any life, no matter what
advantage another may stand to gain.

There is no moment when the rights and claims of
others, whether of unwilling parents, or recipients
awaiting a transplant, would overrule the right to life,

and consent, and appropriate medical care of any human subject, whatever his condition. If there is a true conflict of medical interest between subjects, as may sometimes happen at childbirth, or if a choice has to be made when treatment is scarce, then each must be seen as a party to the conflict in fair terms, and there ought to be no *a priori* assumption in favour of either life. The same basic rules apply here as in any conflict of medical interest. No life is simply dispensable, or simply available for the purposes of others.

The condition of life presents itself to us as an invitation, perhaps an invitation that we would rather not have received. But the invitation gives one option only. It prompts the question: "What more ought I to do for this patient?" This is an open and constructive question, and it admits always of a wholesome answer, even when that answer may be an honest recognition that there is nothing more to be done.

Pregnancy and death are times of particular emotion. Our emotional responses, especially the negative ones, like despair and regret, sometimes lie in an opposite direction to our considered judgement. Negative emotion and clear thinking seldom lie together. The modern world would seem to have accepted abortion as a maternal option, and many people would adovcate voluntary termination when one's own life is no longer wanted. The tragedy inherent in this state of affairs reminds us that ethics is not just a matter of careful thinking but a human task in which an understanding of life and providence is enshrined in a caring and generous society.

The signs of life tell us when life has begun and when it has ended, but they do so, not by prompting a judgement about the quality of that life, but by indicating to us when we can reliably assume that the first moment of life has already come or that the final moment has already passed. Such knowledge is vital to a proper and ethical management of life in the womb, even when it may not be necessary to take extraordinary means to support that life, and it is vital to the proper and ethical management of terminal illness, whether or not it may be prudent to allow nature take its course and to accept the dispositions of providence. The condition of life will help us to decide not what may be done with the patient, but what we ought to do for him. It urges us to create a society and an ethic in which all life is tenderly supported and appropriately cared for at every stage of its course.

4 Consent and life

JOHN IS A patient in his sixty-ninth year. He is of sound mind and a happy disposition. He knows that he is not expected to live more than three months, and that waiting for death promises to be a painful and distressing experience, both for himself and for his two sons. He is a religious man, and he is thankful for a full and responsible life. He wants now to terminate that life, or hand it back to God, and would be quite happy to administer to himself whatever drug the doctor would recommend for this purpose. There is no question of despair, it is a calm judgement based on the inevitable. He wishes only to assist nature in her last service, and to take his leave with dignity and a minimum of commotion.

In the next ward is Anne, aged thirty-six. She has been unconscious for some hours and her death is imminent. Her doctor, wishing to learn a little more about the management of her illness, had hoped to perform a further surgical operation that might have postponed her death some days. He is unwilling to do so now, as he has not discussed the matter with her, and he knows that such an operation would not be of any personal benefit to her. He has asked the nurse on duty to be sure and tell him should Anne regain consciousness.

The doctor's attitude to the consent of Anne derives from the nature of the medical relationship. She and he are equals as human beings, even though the doctor enjoys medical competence and authority. This competence and authority allow him to take responsibility for the management and healing of the patient, with the patient's consent, and allow too for a certain element of risk which may be necessary if the patient is to be helped. Competence and trust and law protect the doctor and the patient in this relationship with one another. But the consent of the patient is essential. No man, it has been said, is good enough to govern another without consent. This applies also to medicine.

What should the doctor's attitude be to John's request? The decision to end one's life is unlike any other kind of decision. Life and time come to us once and for all. We cannot, for all our worrying, add one single cubit to our span of life; but dare we, on the other hand, refuse for a moment the invitation to live?

Moral insight

There are two main arguments of a practical kind offered in defence of life. One is the "floodgates" argument, which suggests that if we allow patients a right to terminate themselves, or be terminated, then we have introduced a breach in our ethical code which would open the floodgates for many abuses, and medicine would have betrayed its task of caring for and sustaining every patient to the end. The other is the "trust" argument, which suggests that medicine must support life always if it is to retain the trust and confidence of patients. If medicine were to become an agent of death, then all medical care would be bound by fear. Each of these arguments has merit, yet each falls short of the kind of conviction that we need on issues as central as this.

Unexpectedly perhaps, the truth about consent is more evident than the truth about life. We would all wish to be consulted, and we do not presume from others what we would not want to be presumed from ourselves. We depend on one another for freedom, support and healing, and we recognise the need to protect one another in our relationships of dependence. The most basic protection is the right to say yes or no. Consent is an essential ingredient of all ethical practice; reason demands it. It is my right to decide whether or not to accept any medical treatment, no matter how well-intentioned the doctor is. It is even more convincingly my right to offer or withhold myself from any service that would not be to my benefit. I am at least master of myself, and of my own giving. We would expect every reasonable person to share and cherish this insight. Consent is a public moral issue, and it is inconceivable that society would tolerate the practices of any who would not agree.

Respect for one's own life is a more personal issue. It belongs to the realm of what we would presume for ourselves only. It could be argued that my own life is the only life that I can end without consulting anybody. What we would do and presume for ourselves takes us beyond the regions of shared reason and into the foundations of our personal and moral belief. There is no compelling argument which all men can share which would prevent John's decision concerning himself, unless it be an argument which recognises that life and time are a gift of God, that they are an invitation from him.

Consider for a moment what the alternative view of life would be. If we were to allow that a decision to end one's life is good and honourable then we have created a completely new option on the challenge of life, an option which would destroy our trust in the providence of God. This is not the place to make any judgement on people who have made such a decision. To propose that it may be good to take one's life is to presume the right to judge life, and ourselves, in absolute terms, to say that life is not good enough, to refuse the human task if we do not like it. We were not asked whether we wished to be born, how could we be? The difference between

existence and nothingness is infinite, there are no
degrees of "in between". To exist is to have been
gratuitously called to being, whatever the circumstances,
whatever the tragedies. To induce the closure of life is
to refuse the invitation, to say that the gift is no longer
worth the receiving. There is no tragedy, whether
physical or moral, that does not lay us more open to the
purposes for which we have been born. To encourage or
support one another in the conviction that it may be
best to end everything now is to betray in one another
every moment that we have been born for, it is to betray
all the moments that are to come, and the opportunities
for oneself and for others that life will continue to
provide. It is to betray the full measure, to withdraw the
cup before it has been filled. The number of years is
not important, but each one is a chance that can never
come again, each one is the only opportunity we have to
live and to respond to life. It is for God to take life, and
it is for him to replace it with himself.

Our religious faith reminds us, "Thou shalt not kill".
Yet we may honestly ask whether this could not have
been known unless it had been intimated by God. Could
it not? Is respect for life a matter of religion? Surely here,
too, we are in the presence of a public moral issue in any
society, and one which hardly admits of dissent. Respect
for life is the foundation for human living, because it is
respect for self.

Consent and life are insights of fundamental importance. They are basic to society. They are not private opinions which we are free to hold or disregard. We cannot be agnostic about them, whatever our faith or conformity. Each is a kind of absolute which everybody needs to see.

Practical decisions

There have been times during Anne's illness when her
consent was unavailable, because she was unconscious,

or because she was incapable of understanding in an informed way what needed to be done. On these occasions, when an important decision required to be taken, the doctor presumed to act only in her medical interest. That is, no other consideration governed decisions that were taken in her regard. What was done was done without reference to any needs other than those imposed by her own illness.

Informed consent is frequently unavailable in medical care. The unborn, the child, the mentally handicapped and the temporarily unconscious are all incapable of giving consent. That fact gives nobody the right to presume consent, unless that consent is to an action or procedure which will be done solely in the medical interest of the patient. Consent may never be presumed for a risk or injury or intervention that is not demanded by the patient's own welfare. We would never presume such powers over those who would refuse consent; what right then could we have over those who cannot refuse? We must seek consent where it is available, and then we may act ethically on what is consented to. Where consent is unavailable, then we enjoy no freedom to proceed, except in the direct medical service of the patient whose consent we have presumed. For medicine to be ethical it must act always in accordance with this insight, and it ought always to lean against policies or procedures, whether clinical or administrative, which would tend to undermine it.

The moment has arrived in John's illness for a decision concerning further treatment. It is clear that he has entered the closing phase of life, a phase which is dictated by his illness which has now passed its critical stage. There is no treatment which will restore him to bodily health. If he were a less perceptive person than he is he would be tempted to lose hope. But he knows that all hope has to be realistic, and that there is no sense in hoping for what cannot be hoped for. He has adjusted the grounds of his hope and looks forward now to a happy leavetaking, a peaceful and grateful death.

What he does not realise is that the months of life that are left have their own promise. Life that is sick and painful is no less human, and need not be less dignified, than life that is well. The days that are ahead beckon him forward with a promise of deeper awareness and a more generous acceptance of life.

It is a mistake to think that the best service we can do when we are in distress is to remove ourselves. We serve one another also when we depend on one another. John has always been an independent man who made provision for himself and for others. He is unfamiliar with need, and with the kind of giving that takes place when you begin to receive. Perhaps he has misjudged his sons. Perhaps he will deprive them of caring for him. To die now would be to die poor; the months that are left are months of promise.

Decisions about further treatment will be based on the fact that he is not going to get better. Therefore the treatment will be caring treatment, and not carried out for the purpose of curing what cannot be cured. Happily there will be no difficulty or misunderstanding in this case between doctor and patient about what is taking place. There will be no temptation to subterfuge, or to hiding the truth; the patient is happy with the truth and needs only to be helped to view it more constructively. There is no need for talk of improvement, when the reality is patently one of disimprovement. There is no need for medicine or procedures which offer "new hope", because John is in calm possession of a profound and real hope that is in harmony with everything he knows.

There are many times when consent and human life hang on a thread, when respect for them needs to be staunchly defended. If the drift of opinion and practice swings against them, the courage with which they are sustained appears as a pointless virtue. Why persuade John to live? Why not make use of Anne? It is so easy to conclude that John has nothing to give. That same conclusion gives value to Anne only because there is something to be taken. It is in the moment when we are most threatened that we need to affirm ourselves. It is when we are most tempted to make use of another that we need to protect selflessly what is not ours.

Precision and flexibility

Not every kind of consent is of value. It needs to be informed and it needs to be free. These qualifications play a very important role, they make the concept of consent more precise, and at the same time they make it more flexible. What is involved in "informed" consent will vary from one patient to another, and from one circumstance to the next. The patient would need to have a basic grasp in simple terms of what is proposed, and some understanding of the significance of this for his life. As regards freedom, there ought to be no evidence of pressure or force or inducement which would undermine consent. Again, precision and flexibility are important. A man can be coaxed without having his freedom taken away. On the other hand, particularly where research and experiment are involved, there can be a temptation to induce some persons with a coaxing that takes unfair advantage of their needs or aspirations, such as might happen with students or prisoners. Special care must be taken to protect the consent of minors and of any group who lack adequate discretion.

There are some things that in a moral sense we are not free to consent to. We ought not to consent to what is wrong. Once again we meet another qualification. Freedom of consent is bound by what is reasonable, at least where other people are concerned. This is more likely to arise where a person refuses to give consent to a procedure or treatment which would protect others.

A patient who is suffering from some dangerous infectious disease is not free to withhold consent to treatment and care which would protect others, even when such treatment would necessitate quarantine or institutional care.

It is essential that moral insight be spelled out in terms of the rights, freedoms and obligations of patients and doctors. Precision and flexibility are necessary if insight is to discover practice and fruitful application in daily life. Moral injunctions apply themselves differently in different situations, and no rule is so inflexible that it always expresses itself in the same way. There is a sense in which all ethics are situation ethics. The ethical or moral judgement is one in which proper account is taken of all the values that are present in a particular instance, and an honest attempt is made to determine the right course of action. Not all values are dominant ones, and some values cannot always be realised. Consent and respect for human life are values which we can never afford to overlook. Difficult decisions will come, but no decision will be moral that does not allow itself to be informed and guided by these two values.

Respect for human life is likewise precise and flexible. Life is not to be prolonged at any cost, nor death postponed when it is due. We ought never to take life directly, nor posit any action which would directly exclude or isolate any human being from ordinary means of support and sustenance. As with consent, this insight will apply differently, but it will always apply, and an honest conscience will be open always to the demands that respect for life will make, even in tragic and perplexing situations. What is at stake is a fidelity to the healing and caring task of medicine, which seeks always to cherish and support the human person to the very end.

What is the caring task of medicine? What is a patient? A patient is someone who is suffering illness. The sufferer may be any age, any condition. In order to help him or her the doctor must learn first to reach in across the barriers of illness, and touch the personality in a way that communicates compassion and care. This is especially the case when a patient is not going to get better. In this situation the caring role of medicine comes into its own. The doctor and nurse will realise that the patient is most probably less experienced than they are in facing death, and knows not much more than they do about what it will be like. We are all novices where death is concerned, whatever the colour of our hair or the shape of our back. Does it matter that the doctor or nurse may feel unsure of what is on the other side? Does it matter when they feel unable to call on religious faith? From the point of view of the patient, surely uncertainty is as good a ground for encouragement as a certainty which would pretend to know everything? The sick person asks only that somebody walk with him the last mile, and that that person offer him encouragement from the resources of his own faith in life. No more can be asked, yet that little can be immense. The patient will go through the final door alone, but he is happy and consoled to know that someone who loves him is standing by. Doctor and nurse are human companions, and it is from a foundation of humanity and companionship that their medical expertise draws its moral strength and conviction.

In a few hours Anne will be dead. Perhaps John might be persuaded to reconsider his position if he were asked to offer his illness and his dying to medical research. This may mean having to submit to surgery and medication that would not otherwise be necessary, it may mean that his death will be made more painful, not less. In this situation the companionship of doctor and patient reaches a new level. We are accustomed to thinking of patients being profoundly grateful for what they have received. Doctors too can be moved by what they are freely given. Professional relationships seek a particular balance between detachment and involvement, a balance which is content once all professional obligations have been discharged. But the enlisting of John for this new purpose reaches beyond professionalism as such. It takes something out of the doctor when he asks and receives the consent that is John's to give. That something keeps medicine human, and may be the saving of professional providers.

5 Turning points

THE MOST DIFFICULT day for Anne and her husband was the day they decided that nothing more would be done. The medical facts were clear enough, there was little more that the doctor could do. He had explained from the beginning what the options were, and together they had systematically explored each of the avenues that seemed to offer hope. Her cancer had started in the womb, and even though Anne had become pregnant for the fourth time, the womb was removed because the doctor knew that there was no hope for the foetus, and there was very little hope for Anne unless the womb was taken without delay. But each avenue turned out to be a cul-de-sac. It was a tragedy. At thirty-six there was no earthly reason why she should have to die.

When a young person dies there is a feeling of helplessness, a feeling of finality. But before death there is a natural inclination to resist, to refuse to accept it, to refuse to believe that it can happen. The drowning man will clutch at any straw. This was why that day of decision was so difficult. That day revealed that the only medical hopes that remained were straws, and Anne faced up to the full dimensions of her tragedy.

It was a day of conflict. What is wrong with straws? Do they not give hope? Is there not always some chance that they will at least delay things? Perhaps a cure will be found? And even if no cure is found, surely at thirty-six every extra day is a victory, every other hour is an hour of life? There was one mercy. The issue was fairly clear-cut. The conflict can be a different kind of agony when the medical facts are less certain than they were for Anne. For her, that day was a turning point.

Joan's baby suffers from spina bifida. As the pregnancy progressed, the doctor explained to her and her family that the baby may be grossly deformed and die shortly after birth, or on the other hand, the deformity may permit of surgical and medical management which would allow the child to live and enjoy a handicapped but real childhood. He advised them that it would always be a special child and its later years would be heavily circumscribed by its illness. Were it not for the knowledge and skill of modern medicine there would be no likelihood of survival at all.

Part of the difficulty is that while the actual condition of the child will dictate the decision that has to be made, it cannot be known now how difficult that decision is going to be. Spina bifida admits of degrees of deformity, and there may be no clear indication of what can be promised and what can not, except in the milder cases, and the extreme ones. The disposition of the parents and the medical advice of the doctor will be crucial should the deformity turn out to be fairly serious. Everyone is agreed that Joan will be least able to face a decision of this kind in the hours after birth, so she and her husband have discussed matters as fully as will allow in advance, so that they will be prepared for their decision when the day comes. They want the baby to have every reasonable chance of survival, and only if it is clear that further treatment can do no good at all, that no qualitative improvements in the child's prospects can be promised, then no steps need be taken to prolong life. It can at least be said that modern medicine often lets us know beforehand what is coming, even if it doesn't make the decisions that have to be taken any easier.

A turning point is created by the realisation that one

does not have to act. One is in a situation in which one chooses to omit; one chooses not to pursue things any farther. The medical options that are left are judged to be insignificant, and a decision is made to accept and make one's own the inevitability of decline. It is one thing to know that death and disability belong to the future, it is another to decide that today the future has come, and that death or disability is the reality now.

The decision is a human and moral one, not strictly medical. There comes a point in the human estimation of things, when it is clear that a personal life-choice is called for, and that medical means are now a secondary matter. The decision that is to be made is made for its own sake, because medicine is no longer capable of playing a critical role in the life of the patient. Medicine has ceased to be an ordinary means of support.

Ordinary and extraordinary means

The distinction between ordinary and extraordinary means is a traditional moral distinction. Ordinary means offer some promise of recovery, where this is likely, or of containment of illness or disability, so that the patient can enjoy an existence in which he can continue to be himself, in which the human task of friend or spouse or parent is capable of being lived. We are obliged always to take ordinary means to sustain life. Such means include proper shelter and nourishment, they include whatever are considered to be normal medical provisions for the maintenance of health and the care of illness, and they include exceptional medical measures whenever these are required for that purpose. Exceptional medical measures, such as major surgery or artificial life supports, become extraordinary when they no longer offer promise of health or of illness tolerably contained. But any medical means that are offered towards the curing of the patient can become extraordinary once it is clear that the patient is not going to get better. At this stage ordinary means are those which will continue to nourish the patient and keep him comfortable, and these alone are all that need to be provided. There is no obligation to provide extraordinary means, and once it becomes evident that they are of no value to the patient, they should be withdrawn.

There is obviously a grey area of decision here. It is not always clear when the will to get better ought to be resigned in favour of the acceptance of illness. Does the acceptance of illness ever become a kind of free option? Are there situations in which illness may be accepted even when some cure that is difficult or hazardous remains untried? Traditional moral theology would allow that there is such an option and that a patient is not bound to choose means that would be unduly burdensome to himself or to his family. For the purposes of medicine and society however, it is better to leave this option to the discretion of the patient, and to presume always in favour of cure whenever this is possible and the contrary will of the patient cannot be ascertained. There is an ambiguity in the concept of extraordinary means. From the moral point of view it refers to either treatment that will not be beneficial to the patient, or treatment that may be considered optional by the patient, treatment that he is not morally bound to undergo.

What would constitute ordinary and extraordinary means of medical care is usually a matter of medical judgement. The distinction is a flexible one and will vary with progress in medical knowledge and expertise, and may also vary from one continent or one culture to another. What are extraordinary means today, may become ordinary in the future. Not everything is practicable in the same way, and what would be acceptable or sustainable in one culture might not be deemed appropriate or beneficial in another. The moral significance lies in the fact that a distinction is to be made between what ought to be considered of obligation and what need not be. It would be intolerable if every patient, regardless of his wishes, expectations or circumstances, had to be taken through every procedure that might prolong his life.

If there were no distinction between ordinary and extraordinary means then everything would be a matter of obligation, and an impractical and intolerable burden would be placed on patients, on families and on hospital services. Implicit in such a situation might be a refusal to recognise the normality and the acceptability of death. Resistance to death loses its rationale when life support has become patently meaningless. Even when it comes tragically at an early age, death ought not to be seen as something to be resisted at any cost. We need to recognise when life is at an end, and the human and dignified response is to meet our dying with calm, and with a peaceful awareness that our time has come.

If there were no distinction between ordinary and extraordinary means there would be a real probability that in some cases even ordinary means would be withheld, while in other cases extraordinary means would be urged where they were out of place. The ready indication of the certain approach of death would be replaced by some more arbitrary criterion, such as age or status, and many whom exceptional means would allow to live would die, and others for whom death is overdue would be pointlessly held in a twilight of medicalised suffering.

The distinction between ordinary and extraordinary means turns on the needs and expectations of the particular patient, not on the nature of the treatment considered in itself. This is why the actual distinction is clearly a moral one. In medical terms, doctors will naturally tend to think of what treatment is normal or standard in a particular case, and what treatments are exceptional. But in moral terms, normal or standard treatment becomes extraordinary means once it has begun to lose touch with realistic expectations of recovery. There is no ethical mandate to provide the same treatment for everybody regardless of their particular needs and expectations. Moral obligation urges us to go the whole way for the recovery of any patient, but once recovery fades as a realistic goal we ought to then recognise that the real needs of the patient lie in the direction of caring only, and of support and strength in the task of dying well.

Direct action and double effect

The most difficult day for John and his family will be the day when he is being helped to die. He has known from the beginning that this day is coming and he has instructed his doctor to advise him at each stage about the progress of his treatment. He has welcomed the support and the care which have made his last months liveable, and he feels no sense of tragedy now that his three score years and ten are nearly complete.

Helping John to die may involve treatment that will certainly hasten his death. Towards the end, as strength ebbs and pain invades every moment, he will need drugs that will lift him from the overwhelming ravages of his illness, and that will give him some moments of relative freedom and relief. These moments may be brief, they may be moments of sleep, when his conscious mind may be mercifully disengaged from the hardship of his condition.

We ought not to scruple about helping people to die. Death is an integral part of life and of human experience. There is no need for it to be one iota more difficult or uncomfortable than it has to be. A drink of water given to a dying man will not be forgotten, either in heaven or on earth. Nor ought we to scruple about the life-shortening effects of pain-killing treatment. There is the world of difference between taking life and supporting it in death. The doctor needs only to ask himself honestly as he administers treatment "What am I trying to do?" He will know instinctively if the answer to that question is "I am trying to kill the patient", or if the answer is "I am relieving pain". To suggest that there is no distinction between these two is to suggest that we can never know when we are doing right, to suggest that we may never act positively for fear of some consequences that will be negative.

There is a very important moral distinction between a positive or good action which may have some negative effects, and an action that is wholly negative and morally reprehensible. It is wrong, for example, to directly take life, but it is good to treat a patient well, even when in doing so it is evident that his life will be shortened. In some medical situations acts may have to be posited which have regrettable consequences that are clearly foreseen. This is the problem of the double effect. If the negative consequences are unavoidable, and if the act is still justified in these circumstances, then such an act may be posited. But an act that is directly negative, whose immediate effect is a forbidden purpose, may never be posited even for what is subjectivly considered a good reason.

This is the reasoning which permitted the removal of Anne's womb. It was evident that if this had not been done both she and the child would certainly die. Hysterectomy is a morally justified procedure when it is medically indicated. To take the womb is not to take the life of the child, even though the death of the child is foreseen as an inevitable consequence. If the operation can safely be delayed until the baby is viable, then it must wait. There will be some occasions when the decision to delay is an agonising one. This is not the place to suggest what ought to be done on such occasions, as so much will depend on the medical facts and probabilities of such a case. The removal of the womb is a reasonable and moral procedure, but not the direct removal of a non-viable foetus.

This reasoning is based on the concept of direct action. Acts are held to have a direct and immediate purpose. This should be revealed by the question "What am I doing?" In this case the answer would be "I am removing a womb; it is a moral procedure and I would do it whenever it was medically indicated, granted the consent of the patient." In the case of abortion the answer would be "I am aborting this foetus. I am taking the life of the child because the condition of the mother gives me serious reason to do so." Many people who favour abortion judge the concept of direct action to be a moral quibble. It is the old question of ends and means. Do some ends justify any means? If we consider all means to be possibly moral, then every act is indifferent and all morality hangs only on subjectively acceptable consequences. The weighing of consequences is an important part of a moral decision, but so too is the recognition that there are some things that we ought never to do, no matter how desirable the consequences might seem to be.

Turning points in life belong to moments when we realise that a whole situation has changed. What were important goals and ends up to the present time have faded, and there is a new end in view which creates new perspectives and orders a new set of priorities. It is important that a medical team recognise a turning point in good time. Much heartbreak can be caused by an indecision which refuses to face up to all the facts in a situation, and which piles up ethical problems for tomorrow by putting off the truth of today. This can happen when patients are needlessly put on artificial means of life-support. It is already too late to start assessing this need when such support has been introduced, except in the case of an emergency when there is no clear prognosis. If there has been no proper consideration given beforehand as to whether such treatment is beneficial to the patient, then the question of withdrawal may create unnecessary anguish for next of kin, and for medical and nursing staff. From the point of view of moral significance, the decision to introduce artificial life-support can be as important as the decision to withdraw it.

The withdrawal of artificial life-support or of means that have become extraordinary is not to be equated with taking the patient's life. To switch off a respirator is not to "kill" a patient. Withdrawal of such means accompanies a recognition that a turning point has come, that the patient cannot be helped in his living or dying by the presence and interference of means whose purpose is the maintenance of life. It is a recognition that this life is beyond maintenance because the end has come and death ought not to be prolonged or delayed.

Turning points in medical ethics belong to moments when we realise that a basic principle is to be applied in another way. The principle of respect for life protects the patient, but it protects him by protecting his living and it guides our care that it may be appropriate to what that living may demand. It may demand that we stretch every resource to bridge a chasm, to resume a journey, or it may demand that we put away our bridges and respect the fact that the journey has ended.

6 Distribution and choice

ONE OF THE troublesome anomalies of modern life is the contrast between those who have and those who have not. We live in a world in which everything seems to be possible, and yet there are so many in want, and in want of things that could be provided if enough trouble were taken to provide them. The contrast between rich and poor is very obvious, but it is only the tip of the iceberg. There is the contrast of opportunity, of education, of affection and of personal fulfilment. Even in the rich countries, there is so much deprivation of affection and spiritual support that for many life seems hardly worth the effort of living.

The reason for this must be that the world has misplaced its priorities It has measured success in categories that make achievement a very costly item. There was a time when the best things in life were free. Nobody wants these now, or at least, very few can afford them because the struggle to keep up and stay apace with society and its demands has become all-important. Unless we can keep producing more and more wealth, all of us will starve. Unless we spend more and more on arms and weapons of destruction, we may be wiped out. The ordered peace where man was the measure of all things has given way to a frantic chase to possess and hold one's own castle, and every demand on the pocket or on the heart becomes a threat to survival instead of an invitation to be and share oneself.

A discussion of distribution and choice in medicine belongs to the same discussion in which we consider all distribution of resources in society. The resources come ultimately from the same purse and the same fund of goodwill. The discussion must begin by facing up to the reasonable demands of every patient, and by asserting our willingness to meet every medical need with an equal sufficiency. This is the only point from which ethical progress can be made. It is the only starting-point which will lead to conclusions that are moral, even when in practice everything may be less than possible.

The distribution of medical care is governed by conclusions which are derived from the ethics of choice. In medicine, situations present themselves in which decisions must be taken and alternatives must be selected which will bring advantage to some and which may leave others disadvantaged. A political ideal, or a constitutional right, might assert that all patients have an equal claim to medical care, yet in order to create the conditions in which such an ideal might be realised, we need to choose which patients and which treatments will be given priority. If there seems to be a contradiction in choosing some, in order that fair advantage may be given to all, then it is essential that we understand correctly the ethical grounds upon which choices may be made.

The problem of choice

There is something forbidding about the concept of choosing patients. It has a ring of omnipotence about it. If there is only one place in the lifeboat and two men in the sea, how is a choice to be made, when such a choice means that one man will be taken on board and the other will be left to his fate? Which man is to be taken? If there is only one respirator and on the same day two infants are born who need breathing assistance, how does one choose? Which one gets the immediate attention and which must take his chance and wait till later?

In the longer term, choices about priorities are made on the basis of careful reflection and evaluation. But how does one evaluate a category of patients? How does one compare the needs of cancer patients with the needs of those suffering from advanced kidney disease? The woman who suspects that she may have breast cancer cannot afford to take her place in a queue. She must see a specialist immediately. The kidney patient in need of dialysis can hardly be told he does not qualify because his home is too far from a treatment centre.

Many categories of patients require expensive research, therapy and care. A host of medical and human factors are involved. Most decisions will be concerned with issues that are not black and white. Routine choices at policy level may lack the dramatic or clear-cut quality of the examples that are given here, but the truths that become evident when we reflect on examples like these provide critical guidance in areas that are grey and subtle. If trust is to survive in the community, then the selection of patients and priorities must be undertaken in such a way as to be understood by all, and accepted as just and fair.

Choice is not made blindly, although the principles of evaluation are such that we must close our eyes to factors that are not strictly relevant. The two infants in need of the respirator may have been born into very different circumstances. The first may be one of ten children, the second may be an only and long-awaited child. Circumstances like these are hardly relevant to the choice of which patient is to survive. Like the status of the parents, these circumstances neither add nor subtract anything from the basic claim of each patient as a person in his own right.

There is only one principle of evaluation where

patients are concerned, and that is the medical need or
indication. This is two-fold. It shows first that the
patient has a pressing need for the required treatment,
that he belongs to that category for whom this treatment
is specifically intended. But it must show also that this
patient can benefit from the proposed treatment, and
that a real promise of health exists. The medical indication would be incomplete if other complications
were present which made the possibility of survival
unlikely or impossible. The medical claim lies in the
condition of the patient and in the realistic hope that
the treatment will give relief. If the disease is too far
advanced for the respirator to provide a promise of
health, then the medical claim to the use of the respirator
cannot be sustained.

The medical indication points initially to all patients
who can be cured. All of these have an equal claim,
and that equality must always be recognised, even when
selection has to be made. Many communities are not in
a position to provide a full range of medical care that
will meet the needs of all patients. Expertise and experience, especially where rare disease is concerned,
are in short supply, and are usually available only in
large cities or in famous medical centres. Yet patients
who suffer from rare disease do not forfeit their equal
claim. And patients who have to wait may be obliged
to do so only insofar as their medical need is one which
can be delayed.

The medical indication points also to all patients who
are in need of care now, those who can be cured and
those who cannot. It is unthinkable that those who
cannot be cured would be disadvantaged by not receiving
whatever care that they can be given, even though
there will be no improvement. These are the most
vulnerable of all, whether they are cancer patients who
are soon to die, or mental patients, who will live on.
How can the medical needs of these be unfavourably

DISTRIBUTION AND CHOICE

compared with those of any other category of patient? In its crusade of healing, medicine must not allow itself to be tempted to forget those for whom there will be no crusade. Our allocation of resources and priorities must include all of these patients and there must be no disadvantage when it comes to dividing their share from the rest.

This same principle of evaluation, the medical indication, governs also our choices of priorities, although its application here is more complex. The elimination of malnutrition and related illness, and of living or working conditions which are prejudicial to health, would take a natural precedence, because they are a direct threat to the creation and maintenance of health in the community.

In the longer term, prevention takes precedence over cure, and the medical effort is inseparable from the drive to displace those causes which undermine health, causes which can be related to deprivation and to indulgence. At this level the medical indication draws attention to many different kinds of priorities, whether it be the eradication of tuberculosis, or the instruction of children in the proper care of their teeth, or the investigation and tackling of the causes of heart-disease and the care and cure of those who are afflicted by it.

The medical need distinguishes the patient and medical priorities from other persons and projects in society, and it focuses on the particular nature of medical demands. It is the fundamental indicator of how choices are to be made. It gives a perspective in which projects for the elimination of diseases and their causes may be ethically evaluated, and it indicates the needs of all patients for appropriate medical care, whether or not they are suitable or eligible for particular treatments.

Because of the problems created by scarcity, however, and the consequent need to make choices, situations can arise in which the problem of selection presents itself with devastating simplicity, and without the refinement of medical qualification. On such occasions the medical judgement leads only to the antechamber of real decision. The medical indication may provide each of the infants with an irrefutable claim to the respirator. This is the crucial stage of selection, when a choice must be made from among those who are eligible, because not all of those who are eligible can be included for treatment. There is no recognised or recognisable criterion for evaluation at this point. All patients who are eligible are equally eligible. There is no way of assessing which infant is more deserving of treatment, because neither is more deserving. And so it is with all medically eligible patients, be they princes or peasants, fathers of families or infant children.

There is only one way forward in this situation, one way which is susceptible of acceptance by those who are likely to be rejected, as much as by those who are likely to be selected. This is the way of chance. This is the only way which gives everybody the same opportunity, which recognises that those who are likely to be rejected and those who are likely to be accepted belong to the same group. All patients who are equally eligible must know that they are equally eligible for rejection and for selection. The usual and most familiar form of chance selection is "first come, first served". Each patient waits his turn and any patient who has begun the treatment is entitled to continue and any patient who has a valid medical claim may exercise that claim when his turn comes. The practical rule of "first come" is a radical and fully acceptable form of selection which is as old and as civilised as chance itself.

The significance of this kind of selection is not so much the element of chance as the recognition that every patient is equal. To sit in judgement upon patients, or to attempt any evaluation of one life over another, whether based on achievement, or responsibility or even handicap, is beyond the bounds of medical and of human competence. The doctor may sometimes feel that he has to "play God" in his role as a decision maker, but to "play God" in the sense of attempting to evaluate one life over or against another would be a kind of blasphemy against his fellow man. The doctor does not "play God" even though the demands of his calling admit him to crucial and agonising moments of practical decision.

The nature of medical care

One of the dilemmas of modern medicine is created by the way in which new and expensive treatment can alter our expectations. When kidney dialysis first became available it was very expensive, and possible only for a strictly selected few. But in becoming available, dialysis changed our expectations concerning kidney disease. What had been up until then accepted as inevitable now became unnecessary. Every eligible patient wanted the new treatment and we all saw kidney failure in a new light. The selected few became a challenge to our existing priorities, and the tolerated incidence of the disease and its consequences began to occupy a new place in our thinking. A quiet killer had become a major issue, and the few who could be saved became a pressing multitude. Our whole deployment of resources was threatened. If nobody need die, why was not everybody being saved? It seemed unethical to say that the issue was one of cost.

There is a special sensitivity in the relationship between medicine and money. There are some things that money cannot buy and if we attempt to market these things, we corrupt them, and we corrupt money as well. Possession of money ought not to create medical priority, and lack of money ought not to be reason for the witholding or delaying of anything that medicine ought to provide.

The patient's need is the need of the sick man. It is a need of support and healing, a need that runs deeper than reward and payment, because the patient is removed from the world of exchange and commerce and is placed, however briefly, in the world of dependence. He is at our mercy. His state of need makes his ability to pay or its absence, irrelevant. The sick man is a receiver, one to whom we give. Money is a secondary matter which is related to the way we organise the payment of our doctors. The same consideration applies to education. The money that passes is related to the way we organise the payment of our teachers. There ought not to be a correlation between individual wealth and the right of a child to a reasonable education in our society.

How we organise the funding of medicine is a practical matter. Fees, insurance schemes, comprehensive free medical services have each their advantages and disadvantages. The point at issue here is the insistence that medical need is prior, and that it alone should dictate access to what we can afford to provide. There is something priceless about the nature and quality of medical care. It is not a consumer product, available for a price. In our society, vast quantities of capital and expensive expertise are engaged in the production and advertisement of medical and para-medical products. It should always be remembered, however, that productivity in medicine is measured in terms of health and sickness, not in terms of financial return.

The material side of medical care is the only aspect that can be properly costed. Buildings, equipment, wages and time allow of measurement. The spiritual or personal side is beyond price. Medicine is a vocation, and it is impossible to imagine a successful medical enterprise that does not consider itself to be motivated primarily by care for its patients. Care cannot be paid for, it can only be freely given.

Ultimately, medical responsibility is borne by all of us for one another. If there were no doctors, we would have to produce some. Society has no right to demand generosity of its doctors and nurses, or of any man, except insofar as it honestly shoulders its own responsibilities to both patient and doctor in a spirit of generosity and of just reward.

A fair distribution

The concepts of medical indication and random selection find their way into the formulation of policies of just distribution. We have to decide how much of our general wealth we will spend on medical purposes, and we must decide on which purposes it will be spent. There are many eligible patients in society, all of them with an equal claim. The medical indication shows what is feasible at any given time, what diseases can be coped with, what needs can certainly be met. The equality of patients reminds us that having made a judgement about medical priority, then we can only proceed along lines that allow the maximum and most practical availability of medical care to each patient. It may not be possible to bring full care to everybody, it may not be possible to tackle every disease with the same urgency. There need not be any contradiction in this, but there should be a recognition that within fair limits we are doing our best, knowing that some will suffer, knowing that by concentrating on one area, another may have to wait. There may have to be a cut-off point, a point beyond which the full and just deployment of resources will fall short of some needs. This is true of employment, of education, of all opportunity. But we must be satisfied that the cut-off point is justly measured, and we must be constantly dissatisfied that it leaves some who are out of reach.

In divising a policy of fair distribution, there are three dangers that must be avoided. The first of these is a tendency to be guided by considerations of societal contribution. There is a natural preference in favour of patients, or of categories of patients, who make an esteemed contribution to society. These would include the gifted, the learned, the wage-earners and tax-payers, and all of those who would be generally judged to be the stable and responsible upholders of the civil and social order. On closer examination, however, it will be found that there can be no ethical justification for such preferences when it comes to the distribution of medical care. Do not the aged become dependent in their turn, and are not children and families dependent on many whom society might judge to be less deserving. The dangers of a false and prejudicial subjectivity would lead the selectors to select only their own kind, and would create a discontent which would destory the trust which is basic to any healthy social fabric. Not only a consideration of merit but a proper understanding of the dignity of every person excludes any kind of distribution on this basis.

A second danger lies in a too-ready acceptance of the existing maldistribution of medicine. The imbalances are evident in two areas. One is the privileged access of some to medical care by virtue of wealth or position. Neither of these considerations has medical merit. The other concerns the drag on medical resources which is already being exercised by our unwillingness to revise our style of living, especially in respect of illnesses which follow from the demands made by competition and strenuous work, and by indulgence. The problem of choice of patients gets a new twist when the deprived and the indulged live side by side and claim medical support from the same scarce resources. It can hardly be argued, however, that patients suffering from diseases of deprivation have a

superior claim to other patients, although it might
seem that natural justice would support such a claim.
The conscience of the doctor recognises only one
claim in all patients, and that is the claim of medical
need.

A third danger is the use of pressure. Many groups in
society can muster an unfair advantage and can wield
power that is disproportionate to their needs. The
distribution of medical care ought not to be subject
to political muscle. There are some categories, particularly the long-term mentally ill and the handicapped,
who would do poorly by this reckoning. Pressures of
various kinds there will always be, but a fair allocation
and distribution will see to it that those who have no
power will not be left untended.

Modern society is a cluster of many interests, medical,
social, environmental. All of them clamour for their
fair share of attention and support. There is no ethical
blueprint by which planners, or taxpayers, or the
electorate can be sure that all obligations have been
justly discharged. Most of the claims on society represent
needs which ought to be met. The considerations
which have been offered here, namely medical need
and equality of patients, are offered simply as points
of essential reference. They do not tell us where the
money is to go, but they do help us to recognise if it
is being justly spent. The very complexity of these
issues underlies the importance of open debate on the
ethical aspects of policies of medical distribution.

7 Problems of co-operation

MEDICAL SUPPORT and co-operation begin with trust and confidence. The patient puts himself in the doctor's hands, and he exposes his personal welfare to him in an intimate way. Doctors and nurses depend on one another in their care of patients, and the strength of their co-operation resides in the competence, judgement and goodwill of each member of the team. It is to be expected that medical relationships may sometimes be subject to tension. There will be different perceptions of the truth of some matters, or disagreements about medical or related priorities. The tension can lead to crisis when the disagreement is such that one of the parties feels unable to continue. This is most likely to happen when professional or medical issues begin to become moral problems.

A bus driver suffers from sudden but infrequent blackouts, and he presses the doctor to renew his certificate of fitness, for the sake of his livelihood, upon which his family depends, and his morale. A patient has become incompetent in a way which endangers others and yet he refuses to recognise or withdraw from this danger. It is a point of professional judgement which touches on confidentiality, the consent of the patient, the protection of others and the common good. A colleague in the operating theatre is under considerable stress at home and is constantly fatigued and lacking in concentration. So what happens when a doctor becomes incompetent, and refuses to recognise it?

There are many points at which professional judgements become moral ones. The use that is made of confidential information is a serious professional and moral issue, and one that grows in urgency as more and more information is committed to computerised records. Another morally critical issue is industrial action. Standards of professional co-operation and the care of patients can be jeopardised by some attitudes to work, wages or duty rosters, whether these derive from grievance or from laxity.

Then there are the problems which are clearly labelled moral. Our society would be intolerant of deceit, or embezzlement or bribery, and professional ethics on these matters are hedged about with the strictest sanctions and codes. Yet temptations will come. A doctor or nurse may be tempted by generosity or by selfishness to co-operate or go along with something of which he or she does not morally approve. Medicine is a discipline in which many motives thrive. Ought one ever to co-operate in the name of friendship, or of pity? Would it ever be permissible to issue a certificate of illness to someone who was well? Would it ever be right to lend professional support to assertions that are false?

At a further level we encounter problems about which there is ethical disagreement, or an absence of ethical consensus. Here it is a question of divergent moral viewpoints, not simply of personal moral judgement. It is a question of two consciences. Consciences differ on the morality of our approach to the use of drugs, particularly in the matter of contraception. Consciences confront one another where there is a question of the manipulation of consent, for whatever good purpose, especially by means of torture. And lines are drawn where the direct taking of life is concerned, notably at abortion and euthanasia.

The relationship between consciences is a crucial issue in modern medicine. It is overlooked by those who would simplify the medical task and who would describe the medical relationship in strictly impersonal terms.

The doctor provides more than a material service, more than guidance that does not trespass on areas of morality. And the consciences of patients and colleagues ought not to take second place to the conscience of the person in charge. To what extent may a person co-operate with a conscience that is different from his own?

Exploring the issues

There are three obvious areas to which conscience must first address itself. These are the moral gravity of the proposed action, the reason for the action, and the degree or type of co-operation that is envisaged.

It is a fact that familiarity and considerations of emotion and expediency frequently take the sting out of moral questions that we live with every day. One of the difficulties in areas of moral divergence is that actions tend to lose their moral significance, and a feeling grows that morality is a matter of opinion, and that the deciding factor one way or the other is a matter of private conviction rather than of moral gravity. Perhaps the idea of moral seriousness can best be shown by taking an example which would still command widespread agreement in our society. The dramatic quality of the example highlights the moral issue. The example is torture.

Is medical participation or assistance at an interrogation involving torture morally permissible? Would such participation be gravely wrong? Perhaps it might be justified by the need to protect the prisoner from injury that would be permanently damaging? Perhaps it might be justified by the need to extract information that would save lives? Perhaps there are hostages waiting to be saved?

But would not assistance at torture be a tacit approval of it? It might lend it some credibility in the eyes of the officers who perpetrate it, or in the eyes of the regime which commands or permits it? It would certainly be taken as a betrayal by the prisoner, who might be innocent of any complicity or forbidden association. It is difficult to see how such assistance would not appear in the mind of the doctor as a grave violation of the dignity and the consent of his "patient".

What about the degree or type of participation? Is it a participation which is necessary to the procedure, without which the torture cannot take place? There is a difference between certifying the prisoner to be fit for torture, thereby committing him to it, and attending to him afterwards and binding up his wounds. In the first case the action depends directly on the doctor's decision. In the second case the action has already taken place and the doctor is called in for what in other circumstances would be a perfectly moral medical purpose. But then the doctor might feel that his association with the procedure at any point, even subsequent to it, lends a certain credibility to what has been done, and to what will be done again. Perhaps the right course would be to withdraw altogether, and dissociate himself from any part in the procedure.

Torture offends against the first principle of medical ethics in that it does an injury to the person. Even where it can be shown that such an injury does not inflict permanent physical or psychological damage, if modern techniques of hallucination could possibly guarantee such an outcome, torture offends directly against the dignity and consent of the victim. May harm ever be done in the name of good? Surely the only ethical answer in this case must be negative. Apart from the damage done to the prisoner, torture has a brutalising effect on the agents, who are de-sensitised at the very heart of their humanity. Furthermore, every experience of policies of torture includes examples of victims who are wholly innocent of any charge and ignorant of information that is sought. Every suspect becomes a victim without court or trial, and every victim becomes an enemy who is expendable in the interests of others.

In regimes where it is condoned, torture engenders a paralysis of moral reasoning. Those who oppose it are labelled as "agitators" and their moral arguments are dismissed out of hand. There is a refusal to see torture as a moral issue in its own right; it is subsumed into a general theory of the good of the people and reckoned to be one of the necessary evils of the modern state. This defensive tendency emerges in situations of moral bankruptcy and morality disappears behind an ideological curtain. Those who are for it consider it inevitable, and those who oppose it are credited with doing so because of their "political" views.

Some will consider it harsh and unfeeling to see abortion and euthanasia discussed alongside torture. Certainly the subjectivities involved are worlds apart. Abortion is often a traumatic experience and it is always a tragedy. Usually the mother is faced with a threat to her whole way of life, her expectations and her peace. Frequently the desire that expresses itself in her mind is the desire to be left alone, to return to normal, to receive the reassurance of her next period. But the period doesn't come. Society is very circumspect about welcoming new babies and supporting mothers. The situation has to be right. And in situations where abortion is freely and legally available, society has fabricated an ethic of convenience which is eager to accommodate a woman's fears and provide a line of last defence where judgement or birth-control has failed. The paragraphs that follow may shock. They are not intended to be a judgement on any woman. They are an attempt to stand outside the sadness, and to offer a simple moral analysis of what is done to the unborn.

It would seem that abortion, if anything, is even more gravely wrong than the act of torture, in that it offends not only against dignity and consent, but also against life. When we stand back from the individual circumstances that can sometimes drive people to take extreme measures, we must at least admit that, objectively speaking, the reasons for abortion could never be as pressing as they may sometimes be for torture. There is rarely, if ever, another life at stake, and there is certainly no likelihood that innocent hostages will ever be harmed by the silence of a guilty accomplice.

Abortion offends against all the principles of medical ethics. Doctors who do abortions may be sensitive and compassionate people, and they presume that they are simply removing tissue. But they turn a blind eye to reality. They rely on a presumption that is impossible to sustain. It is a presumption which must be patently uncomfortable when the foetus is approaching viability. One week it is removed as an unwanted pregnancy, a week later it might have been saved as an obstetric triumph. There is a frame of mind which comes to see the foetus as an object of choice, and the unchosen foetus as a kind of enemy, a guilty party who has no right to be present.

It has been claimed that abortion is simply a woman's right of disposal over her own body, but this surely overlooks the fact that the mother's body is the natural environment of the unborn child and the ordinary means of its support. And abortion creates a climate of moral bankruptcy where those who oppose it are credited with doing so only because their religion forbids it.

There is a grey area between co-operation that is essential and co-operation that is indirect or material. How does one describe the co-operation of the anaesthetist, or the theatre sister, or the doctor who certifies the patient to be physically fit for an abortion procedure? How does one describe the co-operation of the nurse who prepares the patient beforehand, or who assists her afterwards? What of the doctor or nurse who inserts an intravenous solution to induce abortion without going to theatre? Doctors, nurses and students find themselves in situations where they wonder what they should do.

There are two questions to be considered. The first is the question of what they are doing, what is the proposed action. If the action concerned is central to the abortion, without which the abortion could not proceed, then the co-operation is formal or essential. The actions of the surgeon, the anaesthetist and the chief theatre assistants would belong to this category. If the action is ancillary to the abortion, an action which takes no direct part in the procedure, then the co-operation is material or incidental. Preparation of the patient and care of her afterwards would belong to this category. The second question concerns moral witness. Ought the person to be in this situation? Frequently there is no realistic choice here. A student must learn his medicine, and at least at the level of material co-operation, doctors and nurses are expected to comply with normal hospital routine. Apart from considerations concerning his own livelihood, a person might decide to stay and play a caring and counselling role which would be beneficial to patients, or he might stay in order that his influence and example would be a witness of protest or of defence of the unborn.

It is my conviction that direct or essential co-operation in abortion is never justified. A judgement about indirect or material co-operation can probably only be made in particular situations. On the one hand it is said that any co-operation at all lends credibility and moral support to abortion in society. On the other hand, the argument that it is better to remain on in some abortion situations and do what good one can, particularly at the individual level, has considerable merit. Witness to moral truth can work both ways, whether by total abstention or by limited and reluctant participation.

Euthanasia stems from a sense of pity, not compassion, and probably increasingly, from a desire for convenience.

But it is a pity which betrays. It creates a sense of being burdensome and then hypocritically accepts the guilt feelings of those who think themselves to be a burden. The question "What more ought I do for the patient?" could never give an answer that would permit the taking of the patient's life. In the matter of co-operation, euthanasia presents the same problems as abortion, except that to offer any co-operation in an institution which practises euthanasia would run the risk of adding credibility to procedures which would ultimately make all medicine seem incredible to its likely victims.

None of the other areas of moral judgement or divergence partakes of the gravity of these three. Industrial action admits of measurement and the assessment of risk. If there is a critical danger to health or life, then the issue becomes one of grave moral concern and any participation becomes highly questionable. For a sufficient reason, a negligent colleague may be briefly tolerated as long as adequate cover is maintained and there is a reasonable hope that the situation can be quickly remedied. Similarly, deceit can often belong to a grey area of medical practice, where responsible judgement tolerates or goes along with minor breaches, in the continued interest of the overall good. This is not to say that a good end justifies bad means, but to admit that doctors and nurses may find themselves in situations of some moral ambiguity and they may judge that it is more responsible to stay and do what is right rather than resign. They are not justified in doing anything that they believe to be wrong. Nor are they justified if they overlook a coalescence of minor evils which would make a whole system, and themselves, corrupt.

In many of these areas trust and confidence in an overall policy is of central importance. Where there is a divergence of moral sensibility, one can go some way with a colleague or a policy when the goal that is aimed at is generally acceptable to oneself. Where there is little trust, or where a colleague or a policy subscribes to an ethic that is quite different from one's own, then every decision becomes a burden and the decision to stay on becomes critical. This kind of dilemma can present itself for doctors, nurses and chemists, and it can be particularly acute when it touches on treatment that involves addictive drugs and contraception.

A special word on contraception is called for. The first question to be asked here is whether or not one is prepared to co-operate in any policy or to provide any treatment that would include means that one would not choose for oneself on moral grounds. If doctors and nurses are to enter into the moral difficulties of their patients and if they are to be open to the decisions that patients may make, then they must be prepared to advise them as best they can and make any relevant information available in a balanced and sympathetic way. Much good can be done in the communication of accurate knowledge. Knowledge about contraception is knowledge about what is morally significant in a particular case, and that includes a recognition of the distinction between what is contraceptive and what is abortifacient. If a doctor refuses to enter this area then he resigns the possibility of helping and counselling many patients along lines that he might consider best. He does no wrong when he tries to meet the true needs of a patient in the patient's own situation, even when regrettably those needs might call for solutions that fall short of what would ideally be possible.

This same consideration applies to the making available of contraceptive treatment. It ought to be remembered that there is no moral distinction to be made between means that are medical and the "barrier" type appliances. There are important medical differences. A doctor who says he has no business supplying non-medical means might ask himself what business he has supplying medical means when these are for a simply contraceptive and not a strictly medical purpose? This raises again the whole question of the purpose of medicine. There is bound to be an overlap between medical care which is strictly related to health and sickness, and the use of medical knowledge which is related to other purposes in life. Because the doctor is the only person who is competent to advise women on the use of medical contraceptives, the burden of this provision falls on the medical profession. Many doctors tend to be "agnostic" about the kinds of means that patients request. But this overlap between medicine and life ought to be an area of ethical concern. The presence of a medical indication, and the dominance of a health motive, ought to be integral to medical consciousness.

Family planning is a matter of central importance in married life today, and the medical profession ought surely to be taking a lead in the education of women and of couples to a greater awareness of their fertility and the natural management of intercourse and conception. Such an awareness promises a greater personal responsiveness in marriage and a healthy and balanced approach to the planning and avoidance of pregnancy. As in other areas of moral divergence a blindfold descends when it comes to recognising the moral significance of actual situations. Moral conviction becomes identified with ideology or religion. Some who are zealously religious reject the goodwill of those who are open to artificial methods in some situations, while those who encourage natural methods of family planning are often credited with only religious motivation. If a doctor is prepared to judge that a particular method is to be recommended to a particular patient, then he ought to be prepared to make such treatment available or to see to it that such treatment is available. In my view, a policy which would attempt to meet the true needs of each patient, with personal counselling where necessary, is worthy of co-operation and support, when it provides a service that pays full due to the ideals and practice of natural family planning and includes artificial means where these may be appropriate to the needs of patients.

Wider perspectives

It is clear that the doctor ought not to impose his moral views on the patient, and that neither the patient nor society ought to impose moral views on the doctor. Yet there is something unsatisfactory about this antithesis. At a time when the importance of the person in each patient, and the importance of the life and the mind of the patient as a factor in illness, is being emphasised, surely at such a time we should be searching for points of common concern in the moral views and assumptions that we all, patients and doctors, live by. How can a patient share his troubles or his symptoms with a doctor who holds that the patient's moral views are of no account because they are different from the doctor's own? Can a woman be helped by a nurse who refuses to understand the woman's moral feelings? Ready prescriptions, whether asked for or given, may only be half answers, or worse. If medicine is to be personal, then it must enter into the personal arena. To do this, a doctor needs to feel confident about his own moral views, but in a spirit which will allow him to sympathise with the views of the patient, should these be different. Such sympathy requires trust and freedom, whereby both parties, understanding where they differ, may feel free to go separate ways if they cannot reach agreement. And should there be a parting of the ways, it should take place in an atmosphere of respect, with the doctor indicating his willingness and availability to be of help to the person he has come to know and serve. Moral differences do not imply moral judgements about persons.

It will be objected that nurses cannot be expected to enter into the moral decisions of doctors and patients. But any person who is party to a procedure shares responsibility for what is done. This is the principle upon which the courts and the laws of the land operate, and it would be a big step backwards if it were ever taken away. If we have no responsibility, then we have no say. Certainly nurses cannot be expected to decide upon the morality of each case as it comes along, but they must be allowed their voice at the policy level of the hospital, and individual nurses must be allowed the right to withdraw from procedures which they judge to be morally wrong. It would not be correct for either medical or administrative authorities to draw up policy guidelines involving the co-operation of medical personnel, unless the nurses and the doctors have themselves had the opportunity to express and insist upon their own moral convictions. This opportunity and this task calls for a convinced and articulate moral awareness in every branch of the medical and nursing professions.

The argument that controversial moral issues are private, or religious, matters cannot be sustained. Certainly public morality has a validity of its own, and must allow freedom for every citizen to be moral in his own way, with obvious limitations. But areas of disagreement are part of the social scene, and they are matters of public responsibility. We must decide, not just on religious grounds for ourselves, but on social grounds for us all, what kind of society we would like to create, what kind of freedoms and loyalties we would like to encourage. To say that the society we want to make, all religions and none working together, ought not to reflect the value judgements of any sector or citizen, is to fly in the face of what we are all trying to do. The society we want to make has to reflect something of the values of us all.

8 The healer

HEALING IS A very wide concept that embraces tissue and persons. How are we to understand it? How are we to think about the healer? I have chosen to write these concluding pages on a personal note. Anything personal is a kind of belief which grows out of experience. What follows could be true of any journey or any bedside. That, for me, is why it is important. I want to show that medicine belongs to a human context. There is a story, a stage, an occasion.

The North terminal at Dublin Airport is a large hangar-type building used mainly for cargo. On certain days of the year it takes on the appearance of a full-scale emergency. The entrance is cluttered with ambulances of every shape and colour which have been provided by hospitals and hospitallers from every part of the city and beyond. Inside, stretchers, wheelchairs and walking-aids indicate that a unique section of the population is taking to the air. Helpers, nurses and doctors move about supplying tea, encouragement and medical needs. At one end of the hall invalids are being removed, one by one, up a steep ramp and around a corner out of view. Most of them began their journey at around five o'clock, when it was still dark. A few hours of rest had been broken by a knock on the door which announced the arrival of the ambulance man. By eight o'clock most of them have been removed up the ramp and around the corner. Except for the very sick, their mood is one of good humour and anticipation. A few personal belongings are held in the lap as they are carried along: a prayer book, beads and a bottle of duty-free whiskey which has been bought for bringing back home to the friends. Many have never been on a trip like this before, and they aren't going to return empty-handed.

On board the aircraft the cabin crew show in their smiles that they are not yet accustomed to the demands of this morning's schedule. Yesterday it was Las Palmas or Rome. Today they have watched for over an hour as each passenger was carried in and laid in his seat. Should they skip the regulation life-jacket display and the explanation of emergency exits? Perhaps they wonder, as the plane trundles down the runway, what will happen if anything goes wrong? What will happen if there is an emergency landing? Getting these passengers off would be a challenge to any airport that was taken unawares.

The journey is a happy one. The blind, the lame and the halt make very patient travellers. Breakfast in the sky is a treat and everything gives the impression that today they are seeing the real world, looking down on comings and goings which for them had become a forlorn hope. The cool words of the pilot spelling out the weather prospects and looking forward to arrival on time are a bonus for travellers for whom there is hardly ever any weather to think about and certainly no pressing destinations with onward connections.

At the rear of the aircraft are the stretcher cases, stacked one on top of the other. Those on the bottom see only feet passing by, and to help them to eat the nurse goes down on hands and knees. The cabin crew begin to find their feet and provide unexpected services. The gin and tonic of yesterday is replaced by a request to help someone walk to the toilet today. The centre aisle is a cheerful melee of crutches and uniforms, arthritic hips and pretty faces. There is a timely warning before the long descent, and everything re-arranges itself. At touch-down a little of the anxiety of departure creeps in, but when the doors are opened a new army of helpers comes aboard and each passenger is confidently accounted for. It is a moment of relief, the pilgrimage to Lourdes has begun well.

The reader may ask what this has to do with medical ethics. Perhaps the author has at last shown his hand, his concern is really a religious affair and not a matter of practical medicine? But where does medicine belong? Perhaps we can separate tissues from persons, but can we separate the secular world from the sacred one? Is creation religious? If we take away the perspective of God, what are we left with? Sound religion tends to be replaced eventually by heresy. One of the worrying things about modern scientific medicine is the emergence of a new dualism which fragments and impoverishes our perception of man. In its contemporary form this heresy asserts that the healing of the body is an end in itself. Drugs, surgery and the periodic check-up are looked upon in much the same way as the servicing of a motor. As long as the cholesterol levels are right, and the blood pressure is normal, then the person is healthy. But the wholeness of man can never be a matter of correct levels and normal pressures. The making of man can never be a doctoring of tissues snd functions. The body of man is a whole which includes all that his spirit can be. The mind of man is not a magic box manipulated by a spirit, nor by a conjunction of medical and environmental contingencies. And if we are to address one another as healers, then our address must be with all of ourselves to all of one another. I have introduced Lourdes, not to prove a religious point, but simply as an example from my own experience of the interaction of patients and healers at the deeper levels of their humanity.

A place like Lourdes is a spiritual experience, where the body of man comes into its own. The sacraments and the ceremonies are pageants of that other, more real, world to which we all belong. The sick surrender their grief and they discover that around them is gathered a great human family that suffers and prays. The sick and the well pray side by side, each letting down the burdens of life, each realising that here they share for a few days a priceless gift. It is the gift of need. Each one knows his insufficiency, each one opens his hands and receives. The giving comes from God, the healer of man.

Nothing happens that does not lay us more open to what we have been born for. The human task is engaged at the point where the soul is. I think of Tom and Yvonne. He was soon to die, dark, friendly and quiet. A mechanic by trade, he suspected he would mend no more machines. Yvonne was a laughing, pretty, mother of two children. Neither Tom nor Yvonne was more than twenty-five years old. They were in love. They came to pray for Tom's recovery, and came away with the grace that would help them to part. In those days they knew why they had been born. They touched the pith of life and found it good. There were no words to name what they had come to know. To meet them and spend a few moments in their warmth and understanding was to learn something of what we are all born for.

Across the river from the famous Grotto lies a wide grassy field which is called the prairie. The distant sound of hymns and sermons is carried on the air. Overhead the white jagged peaks of the Pyrenees rise up like the poles of a circus tent to meet a blue canvas of sky. Last year, on the evening before going home, a group of invalids spent an hour on the prairie, shaded by a great cedar. One of them found the courage to ask a question which touched the roots of everything. Why did they come? Had they hoped to be cured?

A woman spoke. She was kneeling on the grass, holding the hand of another woman who sat in a wheelchair. The one who spoke was aged about forty and had a sturdy appearance and the colour of health, the other was drained and pale and could have been in her sixties. The woman explained that the person in the wheelchair was her sister, and that they had both fully expected that she would be cured. It had been more of a certainty than an expectation, she admitted, and they had anticipated and visualised the joy of embracing one another after the cure. They had imagined that the press and television crews would be at the airport to greet their arrival home and record for the world the miracle that had taken place. The sisters smiled and held hands tightly. Their faces were embarrassed and shy. An uncanny quietness had descended on the group and all the heads were lowered. No eyes met. Each one was recognising his own hopes and fantasies of the week before.

The woman continued after a few moments. "The miracle has happened to me. I have accepted her illness and her life. Whatever way she is, she is such a wonderful person, and I want only that her husband and children could know her as I do now."

It was an unspectacular climax, yet there was peace in it. A relieved conversation took place as each one said that something the same had happened to themselves. It was like new knowledge, a new way of looking at things. Nothing had changed, yet everything was different.

These are recollections, not of resignation, but of acceptance. The Healer of Nazareth reminded us that life has its troubles, there is a cross to be carried. But he claimed to have come that we might have life, and have it more abundantly. What is this life? What is this abundance? It is an irony perhaps, but to have met Tom and Yvonne, or to have shared the talk of that little group, was to have seen a kind of life and abundance that is altogether exceptional. There was no untoward excitement, no euphoria. There was a simple, loving kindness that seemed to be of God. Perhaps creation was achieving its purpose.

The cross can kill when there is no expectation of life. It can make us mean. We close our eyes to pain and we shut away those who suffer. Like the cross, they are signals of failure. "Has this man sinned, or his parents?" the pharisees asked. The pharisee in ourselves can be tempted to see in the sick evidence of guilt publicly borne. We protect ourselves from the frailty of the flesh. But the sick person is not different from ourselves, he is not less privileged than we are.

Sometimes we make sickness an object of religion. We elevate the sufferer to some sacrificial pedestal, and we try to see in him someone who is better than ourselves. It is the same mechanism as the unconscious guilt, a mechanism of defence and of self-distancing. The sick are seen as people to be cut off from life and pleasure, people who are to be controlled and kept in their hallowed place because we are serving them and doing them good. We see the cross and are afraid. We minister to the cross but not to life.

How easily does the healing task become a lifeless routine? Chaplains, too, can slip into ways in which they serve lifelessly. The very prayers and sacraments that are given to uplift are uttered and consummated in syllables that bear no trace of hope. Oil that is given for healing is rubbed in with little sense of the humanity that is being anointed. Is it because we grow too accustomed to the cross? Perhaps it is because we would rather not look. We are not ready for the kind of life that is promised.

There is an abundance that the cross can bring. It is an abundance that sees life for the first time, an abundance which brings the sick heart alive and sends it out to every moment and every joy. The chaplain, the doctor and the nurse ought not to be afraid to share

THE HEALER

the goodness that God has given them. It is a goodness which becomes an abundance when they have the courage to be themselves, when they have the faith to know that they can heal. It is an abundance that every patient looks for, and none who drinks from it leaves it less full.

The sick remember more than the ceremonies of Lourdes. They speak of the friendship and the compassion which leaves them grateful and moved. They have realised that they have something to give and have felt the strength that comes from knowing that someone they have touched has been helped.

They remember the beauty of the place. Fresh air, green leaves, sunshine and rain are spoken of as if these were the property of the South of France. Those who can walk remember streets and cafes, and a drink to good health. Do we share life with the sick? Do we have to fly them to a far-away shrine to be told that the out of doors and the bustle of life are part of being human? Perhaps we fail to notice a commonplace abundance that we are too busy to enjoy. Can we not properly appreciate the gift of being able to walk unless it is taken away from us?

We are disciples of the Artisan Healer. The sick and the well are the healers of this world, and the well ought never to doubt what the sick man knows is there to be received and to be given. The sick say that those who are well carry burdens as heavy as they do, crosses of responsibility and worry that come of having to fend for family and friend in a healthy world. The sick man teaches us to take up again the burdens of seeing, walking and serving. The healer, whether he be in bed or on his feet, gives of an abundance that he himself has learned to receive. The chaplain, the doctor and the nurse must learn to bring a happiness that is larger than themselves.

> How beautiful on the mountains,
> are the feet of one who brings good news,
> who heralds peace, brings happiness,
> proclaims salvation,
> and tells Zion,
> "Your God is king!" (*Isaiah 52:7*)

The journey home is a quiet affair. People are tired and at peace. Everybody wants to share something of what they have been given, and perhaps there is a little anxiety that the world may not understand, that the heavy hand of routine will snuff out the candle that has been lit. Such fears are never voiced. One gets instead a happy protest that things will never be the same again.

At the North terminal the unloading begins. Two fire-tenders take up positions, one at the outer wing of the aircraft, the other at the tail. The plane is being refuelled for another outward journey, and every precaution must be taken when it cannot be vacated quickly. The plane is already being serviced as the last of the invalids is being carried away. The next trip is to the islands in the sun, and the plane will return at midnight with bronzed holidaymakers.

Bibliography

ANDERSON N., *Issues of Life and Death*, London 1976

BLISS B.P., JOHNSON A.G., *Aims and Motives in Clinical Medicine*, London 1975

BOYLE J.P., *The Sterilization Controversy*, New York 1977

CAMPBELL A.V., *Moral Dilemmas in Medicine*, Edinburgh 1975 (2nd Ed.)

CHURCH INFORMATION OFFICE, *On Dying Well*, London 1975

DEDEK J.F., *Contemporary Medical Ethics*, Kansas City 1975

DUNCAN A.S. DUNSTAN G.R., WELBOURN R.B. (Editors), *Dictionary of Medical Ethics*, London 1977

FRANKL V., *The Doctor and the Soul*, London 1969, 1973

GLOVER J., *Causing Death and Saving Lives*, London 1977

GUSTAVESON J.M., *The Contributions of Theology to Medical Ethics*, Marquette University 1975

HARING B., *Medical Ethics*, London 1972
Ethics of Manipulation, New York 1975

HINTON J., *Dying*, London 1967

ILLICH I., *Medical Nemesis*, London 1975

INTERNATIONAL COUNCIL OF NURSES, *The Nurse's Dilemma*, Geneva 1977

KUBLER-ROSS E., *On Death and Dying*, New York 1970

LEWIS C.S., *The Problem of Pain*, London 1940, 1957

LOBO G.V., *Current Problems in Medical Ethics*, Allahabad (St Paul Press) 1974

MCFADDEN C.J., *Medical Ethics*, London 1967 (6th Ed.)
The Dignity of Life, Huntingdon (Indiana) 1976

NOONAN J.T., *Contraception*, Harvard 1965
The Morality of Abortion (Ed.), Harvard 1970

PASTORAL LETTER OF THE IRISH HIERARCHY, *Human Life is Sacred*, Dublin 1975

RAMSEY P., *The Patient as Person*, Yale 1970
The Ethics of Fetal Research, Yale 1975

SCOTT M., *Abortion—the Facts*, London 1973

SHANNON T., *Bioethics*, New York 1976

Periodicals

The Linacre Quarterly (Official Journal of National Federation of Catholic Physicians Guilds), 2825 N. Mayfair Road, Milwaukee, Wisconsin 53222, U.S.A.

Journal of Medical Ethics (Journal of the Society for the study of Medical Ethics), (Quarterly), The Publisher, Journal of Medical Ethics, Tavistock House East, Tavistock Square, London WC1H GJR